Stunning Braids

Gorgeous Hairstyles for Any Occasion
from Work to Weddings

Monaé Everett

Ulysses Press

Published in the U.S. by
Ulysses Press
P.O. Box 3440
Berkeley, CA 94703
www.ulyssespress.com

ISBN: 978-1-61243-456-8
Library of Congress Control Number 2014952019

Printed in the United States by Bang Printing

10 9 8 7 6 5 4 3 2 1

Acquisitions editor: Keith Riegert
Managing editor: Claire Chun
Editor: Renee Rutledge
Proofreader: Lauren Harrison
Indexer: Sayre Van Young
Cover design: Noah Mercer
Photography: Laila Bahman
Interior design: what!design @ whatweb.com
Models: Emma Sliwinski, Melonie Torres, Olesya Shayda, Tanisha Marshall,
    Difenni Shi, Ekaterina Vygolova
Styling assistants: Shekeelah Keys, Kisha Marie

Distributed by Publishers Group West

Contents

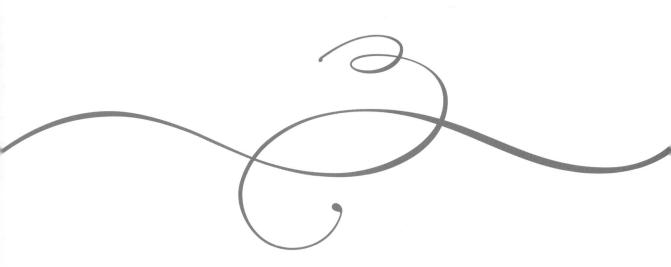

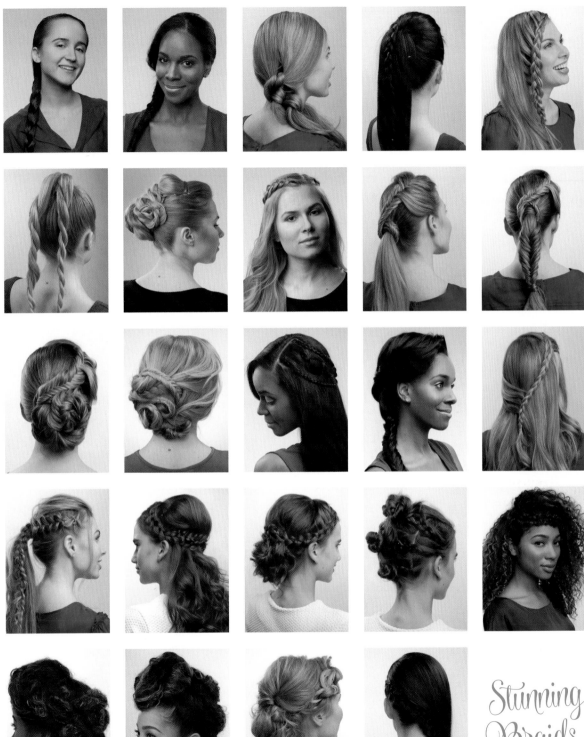

Stunning
Braids

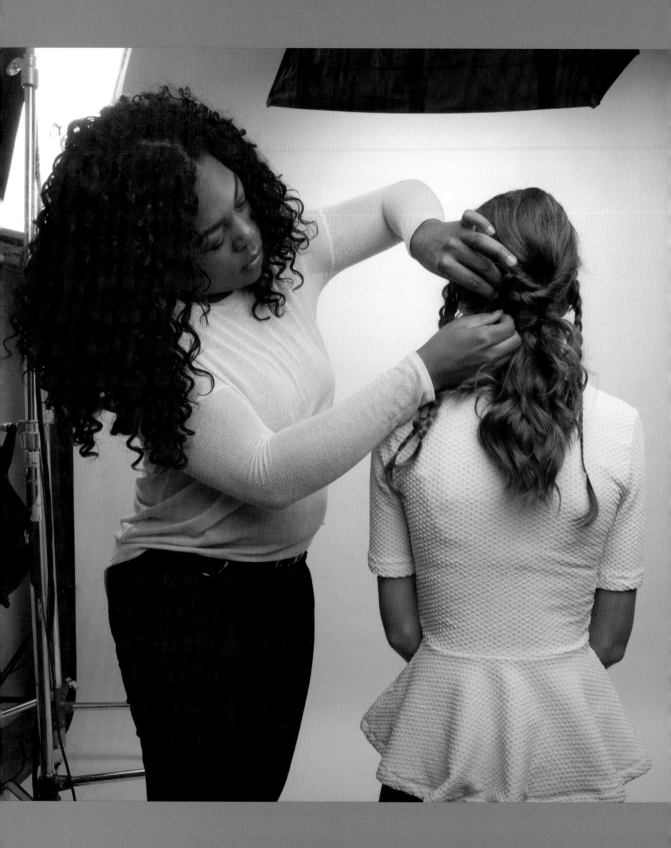

Introduction

Hello, beauties! My name is Monaé Everett and I'm your personal hair guide, here to help you navigate the beautiful world of braiding. Fishtails, Dutch braids, updos, curls, waves, sleek, and gorgeous: I've got you covered. For beginner or advanced braiders, *Stunning Braids* is the right book if you're looking for a unique hairstyle that is guaranteed to turn heads and make an impression.

I absolutely adore braided hairstyles. I started braiding hair as a little girl, giving my baby dolls braided hairdos. Since then, I've become a professional celebrity hairstylist and a braiding teacher. My passion for braids knows no end; I've also created multiple braiding tutorials on YouTube.

What I love about braiding is that it can be as simple or complex as you make it. Because of this, the book is divided into two sections: basic braids and advanced braids. The basic braids keep it simple, introducing some looks that utilize some of my favorite standard braids like the Basic Fishtail and the Three-Strand Twist. The advanced braids take these braids to the next level by mixing and matching some of these different techniques. You'll combine the French Braid and the Basic Fishtail, the Fringe Lace Braid and the Dutch Braid. Before you know it, you'll be at professional status! There are braids for everyday wear, weekend hangouts, music festivals, work, proms, and weddings. Choose a style that fits your personality and get creative!

I've also included some introductory material with some of my must-have products and styling tools you'll need to get started. As another bonus, I've also included some information on how to best prep different hair textures before styling. However, I encourage everyone to embrace their natural texture when it comes to these styles!

Let's get started.

—Monaé

Chapter 1
Styling Equipment

Before we dive into our fabulous braiding styles, we need to talk about the tools you'll need to get started. Throughout this book, I'll reference different brushes, clips, products, and styling tools that tame those locks and make for effortless styling. The following pages have a breakdown of some of my favorites: from my trusty rat tail comb, perfect for sectioning and smoothing the hair, to my tourmaline ceramic flat iron, great for straightening and curling. I highly recommend you invest in a few of these basics, especially the equipment that fits the hair color and texture that you're styling. You shouldn't have any trouble finding these at your local beauty supply store or online. Happy shopping!

HAIR BRUSHES

A. Styling brush: Great for heat styling and use with a blow-dryer. Provides maximum grip and control. The hard rubber will not burn.

B. Paddle brush with ball-tipped nylon bristles: A rectangle-shaped brush used to direct the hair. The nylon bristles increase blood circulation.

C. Grooming brush with natural bristles and nylon pins: An oval-shaped brush with each single nylon quill surrounded by a natural boar bristle. This is ideal for smoothing.

D. Mini styling brush: For use with a blow-dryer when focusing on smoothing the hair line.

E. Hard rubber rat tail comb: A heat-resistant comb that helps when using hot tools.

F. Wide-tooth comb: Excellent for detangling hair.

G. Rat tail comb: Best for sectioning hair, styling, and back combing hair.

H. Styling rat tail comb: Great for the final touches of a style.

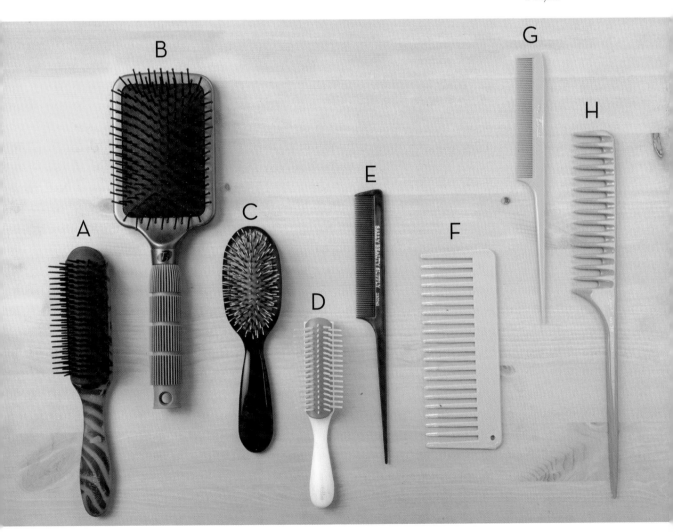

TIES, CLIPS, AND PINS

Hair Ties

A. Bungee elastic: Allows for a custom-fit ponytail, no matter the hair fullness or texture.

B. Large elastic hair tie: Holds large sections of hair and are best for ponytails. They cause less stress on hair than rubber bands.

C. Large rubber bands: An alternative for elastic hair ties.

D. Small rubber bands: Good for small sections of hair.

E. Small, clear rubber bands: Ideal for small sections of blonde hair.

Clips

F. Single-prong clips: Adds texture to hair or holds small sections of hair.

G. Double-prong clips: Holds a small section of hair or roller in place.

H. Spin pins: Holds hairstyles in place, especially buns and chignons. These are the perfect alternative for multiple bobby or hair pins.

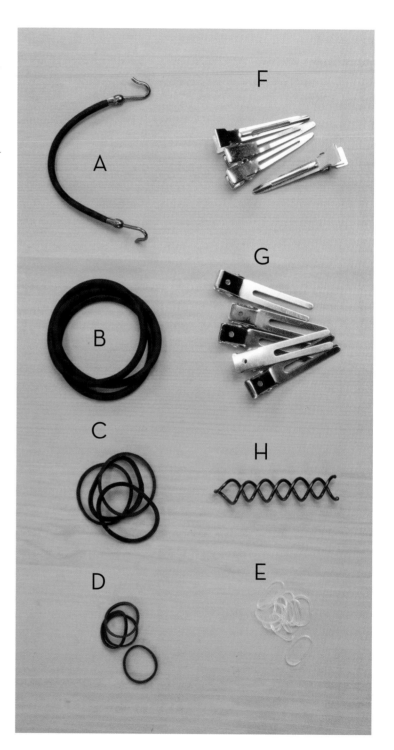

Pins

Braids are typically pretty resilient, but pins are crucial to keeping hair in place, especially updos. Narrow bobby pins work great for securing the base of a style, while the wider-mouth hair pins pin together different sections of a look to create a finished style.

I. Long, blonde bobby pins: Provide a secure base for wide updos. These are especially good for blonde hair.

J. Long, blonde hair pins: Keep detailed hairstyles in place. These hair pins are used for detailed blonde hairstyles.

K. Blonde hair pins: These hair pins are my favorite choice for pinning the strands of a braid in place and into an updo.

L. Bronze bobby pins: Perfect for light brunettes and redheads.

M. Brown bobby pins: Provide a stable base for updos and other styles. These also work well for light brunettes and redheads.

N. Long, black bobby pins: Ideal for dark hair.

O. Long, black hair pins: Pin small sections of hair for creating more detail within the style. Think messy buns.

P. Black hair pins: Great for teased styles. These hair pins are the most commonly used hair pins.

Q. Black bobby pins: Offer a secure base for any style and ideal for dark hair. These are the most commonly used bobby pins.

R. Mini black bobby pins: Secure tiny sections of hair. These work wonders at smoothing the hairline or nape.

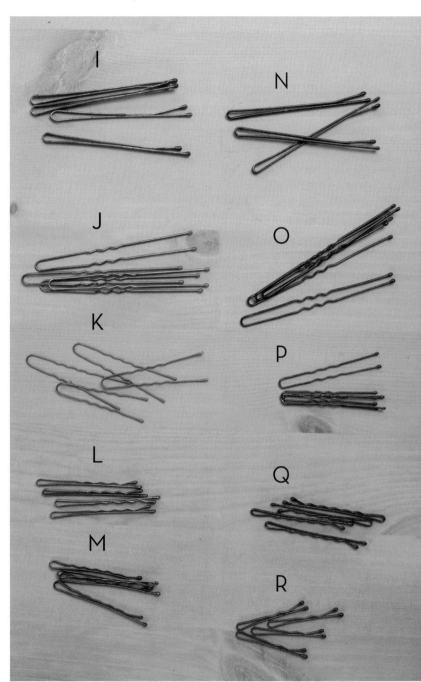

PRODUCTS

A. Maximum hold hair spray: Gives the strongest hold and fights frizz, so you can truly "spray it and forget it."

B. Anti-frizz polishing milk: My favorite product to use when braiding. It fights frizz and dries without flaking.

C. Thermal setting spray: Applied to wet hair before a blow-dry. It's a heat protectant and helps the hair to hold the style longer.

D. Gel: Works best on wet hair. It also helps the hairstyle to set into place and can be used without a blow-dryer.

E. Brushable hair spray: Your best friend in hairstyling. It can be used throughout styling on dry hair. If the style changes, just brush out the hair.

F. Texture powder: Creates texture and works awesomely with braids.

G. Mousse: Added to wet hair to create volume and style memory.

H. Volumizing spray: Used on either wet or dry hair, but creates more fullness when blow-dried.

I. Serum: Increases shine and reduces frizz on either wet or dry hair.

J. Spray serum: Finishes a look when styling is complete.

K. Gel for curly hair: Provides better curl definition.

L. Leave-in conditioner: Offers moisture and heat protection.

M. Styling cream: Applied to dry hair to add moisture and smooth hair when styling.

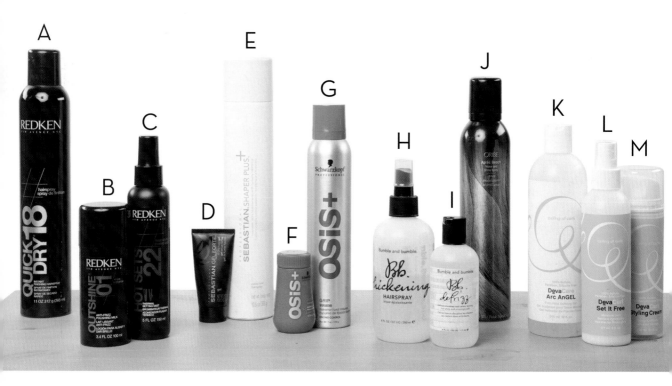

STRAIGHTENERS AND DRYERS

A. Tourmaline ceramic 1-inch flat iron: Straightens and curls hair. I highly recommend investing in a good ceramic straightener for the best effect.

B. Tourmaline ceramic 1½-inch curling iron: Creates large waves.

C. Tourmaline ceramic 1-inch curling iron: Produces different size curls and waves. This is the most versatile of all curling iron sizes.

D. Tourmaline ceramic ¾-inch curling iron: Shapes tight curls and can be used on short hair.

E. Ceramic blow-dryer with negative ions: Dries hair fast, reduces frizz, and adds shine. This is another great investment for beginner and advanced stylists!

A   B   C   D   E

Chapter 2
Braiding Preps

Now that you've got all the tools for the job, it's time to prepare the hair you'll be working with. Whether you're styling on yourself or on someone else, certain styles will look better if you prep the hair before you start braiding. This is particularly true of partial updos, where loose hair is just as important as braided hair, but also to give hair the right texture. For example, my curly haired beauties might want to consider using a flat iron to create a smoother base before starting sleeker styles. Or my straight-haired pretties might add some curls for more volume and texture in their braid. The following pages outline my favorite braiding prep styles, and each braid has my advice for which prep may work best. Feel free to experiment and find your favorite!

QUICK AND EASY DETANGLING

For a no-fuss hairstyle, look no further! This is the simplest way to prep hair for braiding and it's perfect for all hair textures. Just grab a spray bottle or jump out of the shower and start braiding.

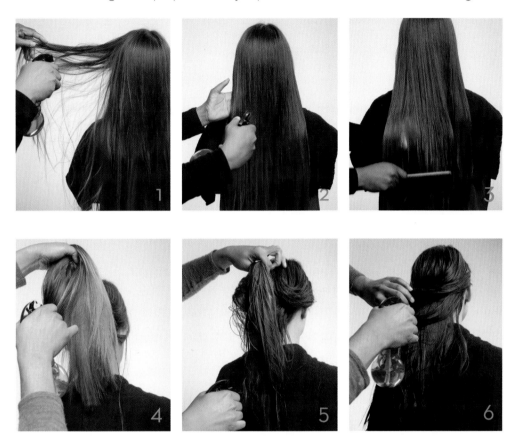

1: Using a spray bottle filled with water, dampen hair. **2:** Start spraying at the roots to keep from using too much water. **3:** Take a moment to comb through hair with a wide-toothed comb, making sure that the water is evenly distributed and the hair detangled. **4:** Gather hair into a ponytail and spray ends. **5:** Once ponytail is damp, make sure entire head of hair is damp. **6:** Spray any remaining dry strands.

TIP: Use a towel around the neck when spraying. Be careful of water that may drip onto the floor.

LARGE ROMANTIC CURLS

The perfect foundation for most partial braids, these effortless-looking waves give hair additional body and bounce when hair is left down. It's easier to create these romantic curls on longer lengths of hair, and it's one of my favorite prep techniques. This quick set is done with a 1½-inch curling iron.

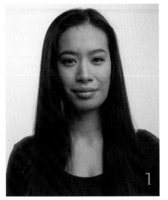 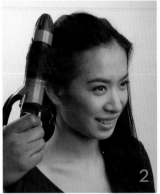 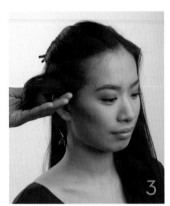

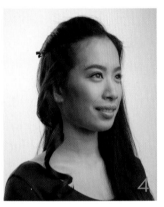 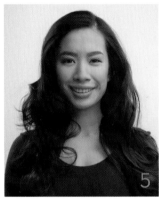

1: Detangle damp hair with a wide tooth comb. Apply volumizing mousse and thermal setting spray. Blow-dry. **2:** Separate a 1½-inch-wide, vertical section of hair. Using a 1½-inch curling iron, clamp hair around curling iron, direct hair away from face. **3:** Hold for 10 seconds, then release. **4:** Pin hair into place. Repeat. **5:** Once hair has cooled, remove pins and spray with a serum and holding spray. Finger tousle or brush out curls.

TIP: Make sure sections are the same width as the curling iron. Curl closer to the scalp for longer-lasting curls.

TEXTURED WAVES

Transform boring, straight hair into fun, bouncy curls with this textured look. This prep is great for any style you chose, especially partial updos that will showcase these lovely ¾ inch waves.

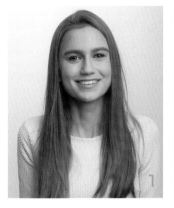
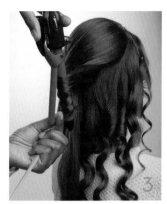
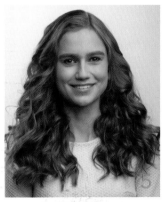
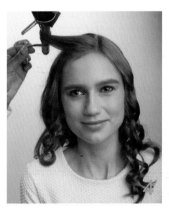
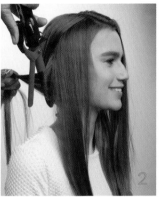

1: Detangle dry hair with a paddle brush. **2:** Using a ¾-inch curling iron, curl a 2-inch vertical section of hair. **3:** Starting a few inches away from the scalp, wrap hair around curling iron. Twist while wrapping. Hold for 10 seconds, then release. Repeat. **4:** For a modern look, direct curls away from the face. **5:** After all of the hair is curled, spray with a brushable holding spray and brush to soften the look.

TIP: Apply a volumizing mousse before blow-drying hair to increase curl memory.

FLAT-IRON CURLS

Flat-iron curls are the easy, all-in-one prep solution for any hair texture. Whether coaxing curls out of dead-straight locks or taming unwieldy curly and coarse hair, this prep offers smooth hair, added shine, and extra bounce for all!

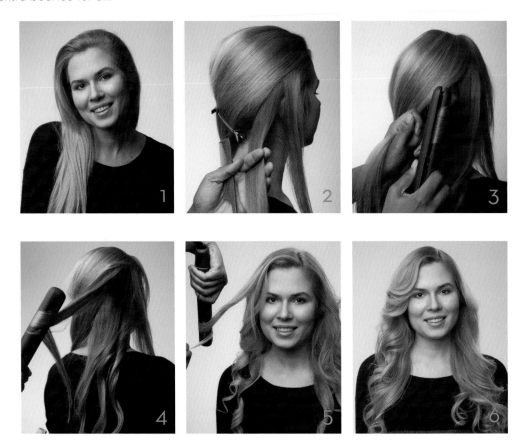

1: Apply volumizing mousse to damp hair. Blow-dry, detangle, and spray with thermal setting spray and holding spray. **2:** Separate a vertical section of hair the same width as your flat iron (1-inch-wide sections shown). **3:** Place section in flat iron, close, turn to the side, and slide down the length of the hair. Repeat. **4:** For a tighter curl, turn the flat iron twice. **5:** For a fashionable and modern look, curl away from the face. **6:** Finger tousle when finished.

DIY FLAT-IRON CURLS

With a few moments and your trusty flat iron, this versatile style can be mastered anytime, anywhere.

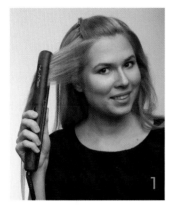 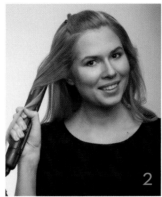 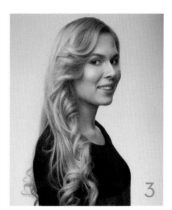

1: Separate a vertical section of hair the same width as your flat iron. **2:** Place section into flat iron, close, twist away from the face, and glide down the length of your hair. **3:** Repeat.

THE SUPER-SMOOTH SOLUTION

Whether your hair is curly, kinky, or wavy, this prep can handle it. Super smooth, straight, and silky, this is best for showing off some of the more detailed braids.

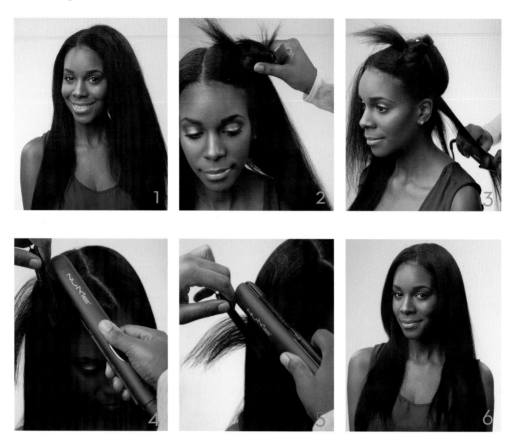

1: Apply leave-in conditioner, mousse, and serum. Blow-dry hair completely and spray with a thermal setting spray. **2:** Divide hair into 4 sections. **3:** Take a 1-inch horizontal subsection and lift with a hard rubber comb. Place hair inside flat iron ⅛-inch from the roots, close, and move through hair. **4:** The comb remains in front of the flat iron to hold hair in place. **5:** If done correctly, only one pass is needed. **6:** Repeat until all hair is straight.

SOFT CURLS

What's the perfect balance of straight and wavy hair? Soft curls. This prep uses a 1-inch curling iron to give boring straight hair a touch of volume, body, and bounce, adding texture and fullness to larger braids.

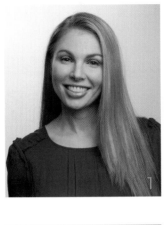 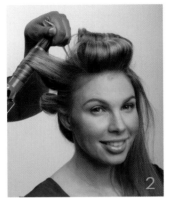 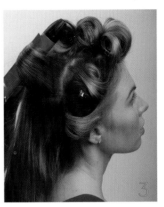

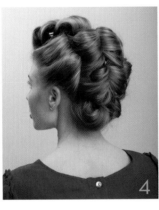 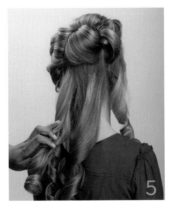 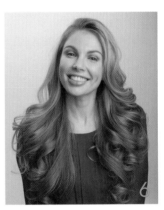

1: Apply mousse. Blow-dry hair using a round or flat brush. Spray hair with thermal setting spray. **2:** Beginning at the crown of the head, select 1-inch-wide vertical sections. Wrap section around the 1-inch curling iron. Release and clip in place to cool. **3:** Continue around the head, curling sections close to the root. **4:** Allow curls to cool completely. **5:** Release clips. Finger tousle, comb, or brush curls out. **6:** Continue on to braiding!

TIP: This prep can be used on curly and course hair after hair has been straightened.

Chapter 3

Basic Braids

Let's get started! Welcome to Braids 101. For newbies and those that need a refresher on the basic braids, try out some of these styles before graduating to the advanced braids. I'll be introducing the looks you're probably familiar with, like the Three-Strand Braid and the Basic Fishtail, as well as a few of my favorites, like the Knot Braid and the Three-Strand Twist. All of the styles in this book include some variation of these classic braids, and many can be swapped or alternated as you customize a style. Once you master the main braid in each of these styles, you'll be ready to take on even the most elaborate updo. Remember: practice makes perfect. Keep at it and it will become easier each time!

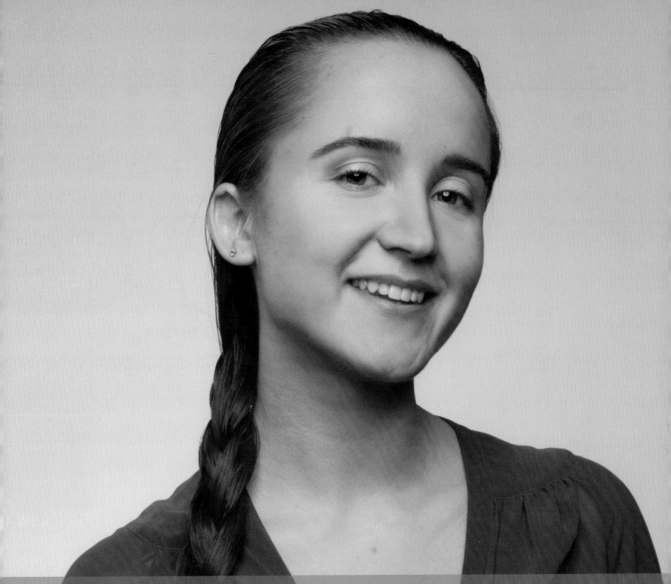

Three-Strand Braid

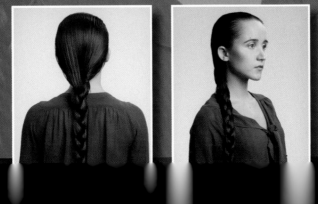

The mother of all braids, this basic style is known as the Three-Strand Braid or plait. This technique has been around for centuries, used by many different cultures around the world, and is probably the braid you're most familiar with. It's a simple way to keep hair out of your face while you're running errands and doing chores, as well as a simple way to style your hair when you're in a pinch. As an added bonus, this braid will hold until you're ready to unravel it.

It's a good idea to learn this technique as a stepping-stone into the more complicated styles. All of the other braids in this book are actually a variation of this braid. Once you've mastered the Three-Strand Braid, you're already halfway to becoming a braiding pro.

I recommend trying this with wet hair. You can definitely do this style with dry or curly hair, but wet hair will help you avoid flyaways, keep hair secure, and make it more manageable. Braiding wet hair is also a great way to make some no-fuss waves. Once hair is dry, simply undo the braid and you'll have easy, no-heat waves.

TIPS FOR PREPPING

This is by far one of the simplest hair preps. After washing hair, use the leave-in conditioner of your choice to comb through and detangle hair. To keep hair damp, use a spray bottle filled with water.

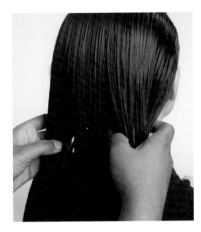

1: Separate hair into three equal strands. Hold the left strand in the left hand, the right strand in the right hand.

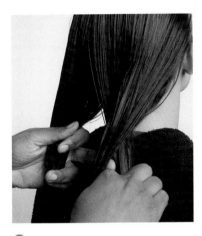

2: Move the right hand strand over the center strand. This becomes the new center strand.

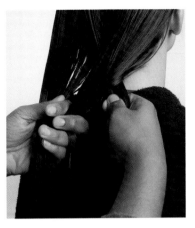

3: Take up the new center strand in the left hand, along with the left strand. **TIP:** Hook the center strand with a middle finger to keep sections separate.

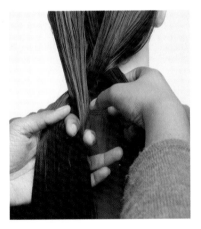

4: Pass the farthest left strand to the right hand, crossing over the center strand. It is now the new center strand.

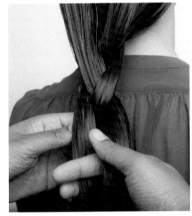

5: Continue this pattern, alternating right over center, left over center. The center strand will move the most often.

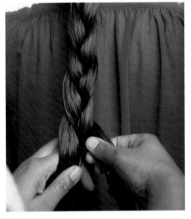

6: It is important to have a firm grip while braiding to keep it even and secure.

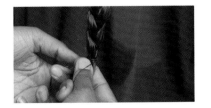

7: Secure the ends with an elastic band. Try black bands on brunettes, clear bands on blondes, and brown bands on redheads.

TIP: Use a gel while braiding to create waves in loose hair when dry.

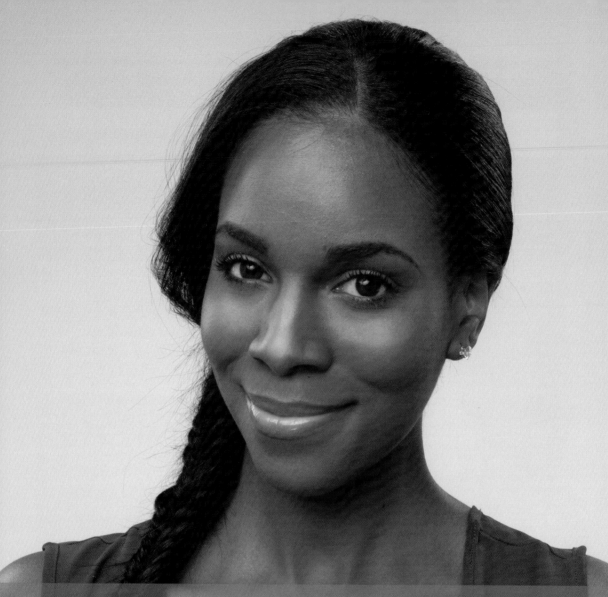

Basic Fishtail

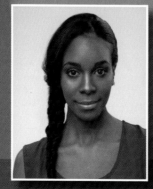
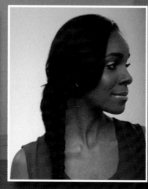

This is the braid that will take you from an amateur to a braiding professional. The Basic Fishtail is one of the most coveted braiding skills, but I promise that you'll be able to handle it. Once you master this braid, it'll open the doors for so many different styles and variations.

Personally, I love to create this look on wavy or straight hair. Straighter hair lends more detail to the intricate elements of the braid. The smaller the pieces you take, the more precise the braid stitches will look. While braiding, make sure that you don't pick up pieces that you just crossed over, or else it won't have the same effect. You'll impress your friends, dates, parents, local barista, and pretty much everyone wherever you go, who will want to know how you did it. And, despite its delicate look, this braid will last until you decide to take it out.

TIPS FOR PREPPING

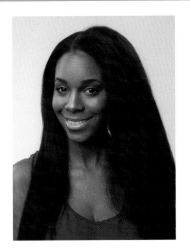 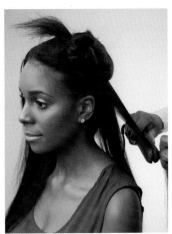 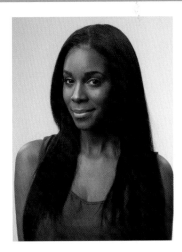

The Basic Fishtail can be created on straight, wavy, or loosely curled hair. For more detail, use straighter hair. Blow-dry the hair straight with mousse, thermal setting spray, and a flat styling brush. Use a flat iron to create extra-straight locks.

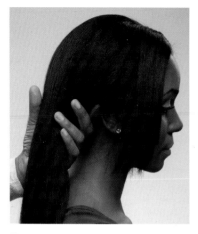

1: Section out fringe. Brush remaining hair to one side and gather into a ponytail.

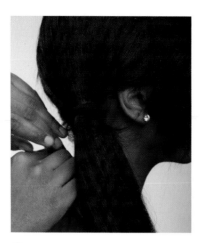

2: Secure the ponytail with a hair-colored elastic band.

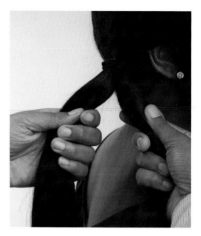

3: Divide the ponytail into two equal sections. Apply a small amount of serum to smooth hair and reduce flyways.

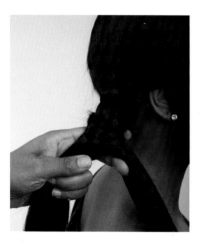

4: Take a piece from the back of the left section around and over the left section, and place it into hair of the right section.

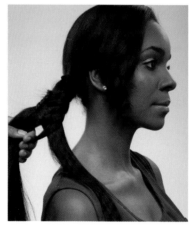

5: Take a piece from the back of the right section around and over the right section, and place it into hair of the left section.

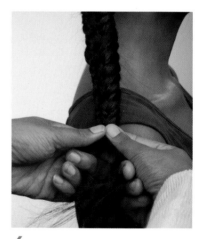

6: Repeat, alternating left and right, and watch the beautiful fishtail pattern form. Make sure to hold each section firmly.

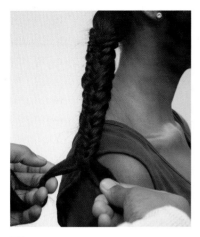

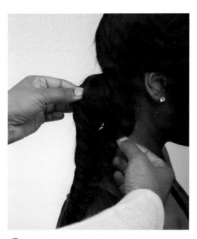

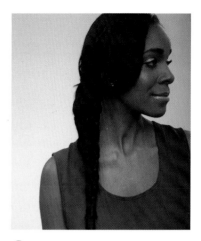

7: Stop braiding a few inches from the ends. Hold the bottom of the braid with a clip.

8: Loosen the fishtail by gently pulling on the outside of the braid. This is called pancaking. It creates more width and texture, making the braid look more fashionable.

9: Remove the clip from the bottom of the braid. Instead of using an elastic, spray it with super-hold spray.

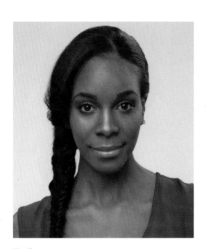

10: Backcomb the ends of the braid to secure it. If bangs are long enough, wrap them around the elastic at the base of the braid. Finish the look with a spray serum.

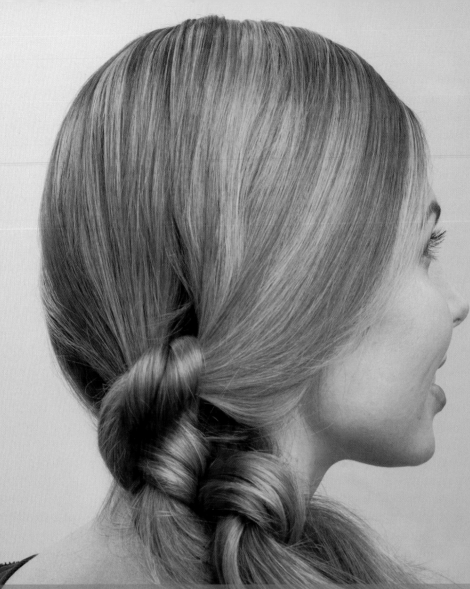

Knot Braid

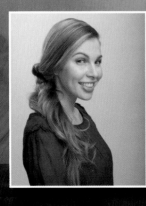
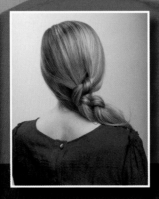
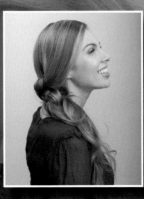

Take up your armor with the chainmail-inspired, quick-and-easy Knot Braid. This is one of the simplest styles possible. If this is your first foray into the world of braiding, I recommend starting here! This is a great introduction to the creativity of braids. Trust me when I tell you that you'll be able to pick this one up in no time at all.

This style is for everyone! It doesn't matter if you're a curly, coily, or straight-haired girl, give this beginner braid a whirl. Feel free to change up your part here and try something new; I always feel a deep side part will make your style appear more sophisticated. This look channels your inner warrior to tackle the toughest of everyday battles, even if it's just finally hunkering down and doing your laundry. This look will definitely last on the battlefield...or a day at class or the office.

TIPS FOR PREPPING

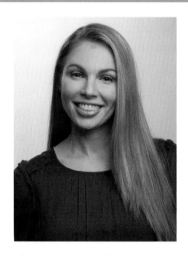 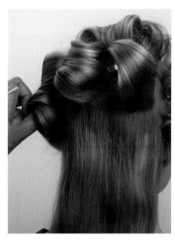 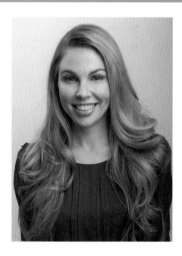

This style works for all hair types, so prepping is really a personal preference. Large, loose curls give this model's straight hair more body and bounce. Hair was curled in 2-inch sections with a 1-inch tourmaline curling iron and clipped into place to cool.

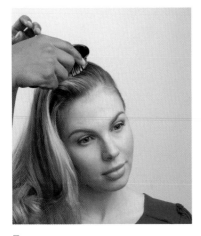

1: Detangle hair and brush it to the right, as if you were making a side ponytail. Add anti-frizz milk for shine and to reduce flyways.

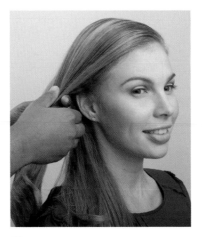

2: With the hair on one side, separate hair into two sections by making a horizontal division behind the right ear. Take the top section and separate it into two strands. Hold one strand in each hand.

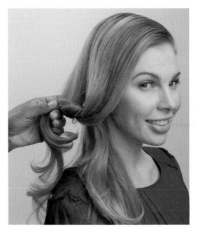

3: Take the hair in the left hand under, then over the hair in the right hand.

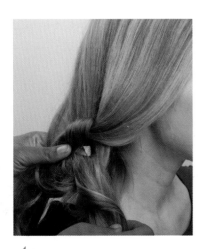

4: This is exactly the same as the first step in tying a shoe. After the sections have crossed, add hair from the bottom to both sections. Repeat step 3.

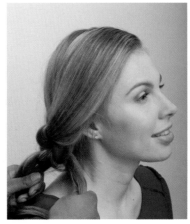

5: Pull on both sections to secure knots. The chain link pattern is starting to form!

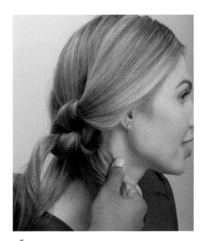

6: Tie the hair one more time for a more secure hold. If hair allows, this extra chain link adds detail.

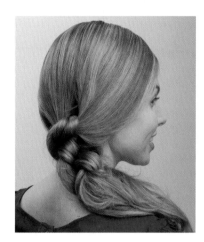 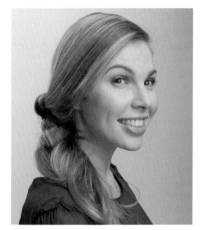

7: Once the three chain links are in place, secure any loose hairs with bobby pins or hair pins.

8: To make a really stand-out look, finish with a shine serum and holding spray.

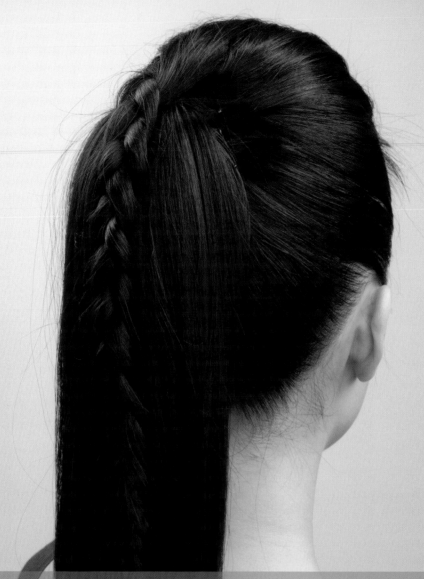

Simple Braided Pony

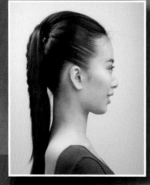

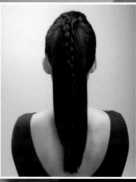

"Less is more." I think this braid perfectly embodies that saying. This super-simple braid is just your basic Three-Strand Braid (page 17), but it has a huge impact as the centerpiece for this style. The Three-Strand Braid is pinned into a high ponytail, offering a super-high-end, chic attitude. The braid can be switched out for different braid techniques; a Basic Fishtail (page 20) or Knot Braid (page 24) would work really well here (and would be just as easy).

The Simple Braided Pony can be done on most hair types, but I especially love the way this looks on straight hair. Too much texture here is distracting and takes focus away from the braid. I highly recommend using a flat iron to get the straightest hair possible. Be sure to use product here. Anti-frizz products will be your best friend when it comes to taming flyaways that threaten the silkiness of this look. Once you've smoothed down the hair, you can expect this look to last the entire evening. Wear this sleek, high ponytail when you get cocktails with the girls or during your next night out on the town.

TIPS FOR PREPPING

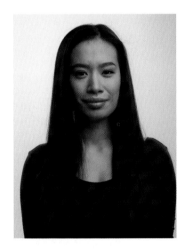 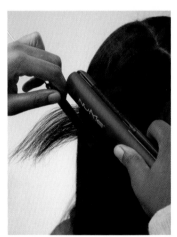 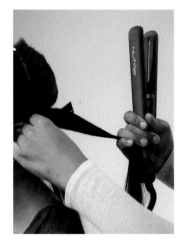

For the super-sleek look of this style, blow-dry hair straight with a thermal setting spray, gel, and a flat styling brush. Flat iron if needed. If hair is dry, bypass the blow-drier and simply flat iron straight.

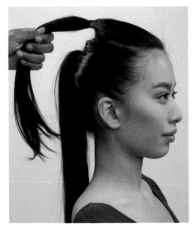

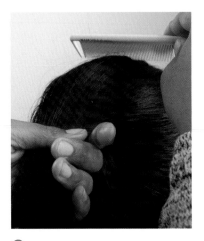

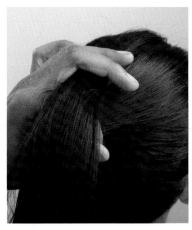

1: Create a 3 x 3-inch section of hair at the front crown of head. Gather into a ponytail and secure with an elastic band. Gather the rest of the hair into a high ponytail and secure with an elastic band.

2: Remove the top elastic. Backcomb the gathered crown pony with a rattail comb and smooth the top layer of hair. Use a brushable hair spray to smooth hair at the hairline.

3: Allow the backcombed hair to lie over the ponytail. Keep hair gathered in hand as a ponytail.

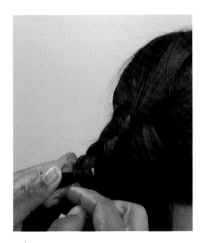

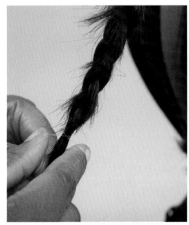

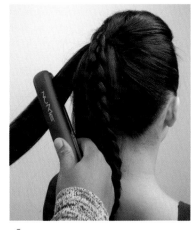

4: Once top ponytail is centered, begin a standard Three-Strand Braid and continue until you reach the ends of the hair.

5: Don't worry about strands of hair that may stick out of the braid. This tends to happen more when hair has been flat ironed straight. Secure the end of the braid with a clear plastic band.

6: Bobby pin the base of the braid to the base of the ponytail to keep secured in the center. To make the ponytail super sleek, apply serum and hair spray, then flat iron to remove extra texture.

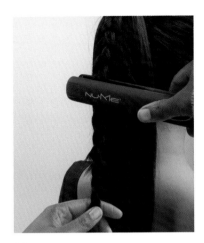

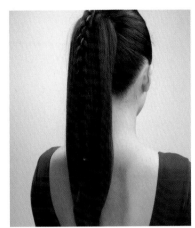

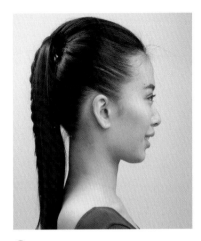

7: Run the braid through the flat iron, avoiding the clear plastic band at the ends. This will tame flyaways.

8: Use serum, hair spray, or an edge tamer to smooth the hairline. For maximum impact, this style must be neat.

9: The look is complete! Finish with hair spray, if needed.

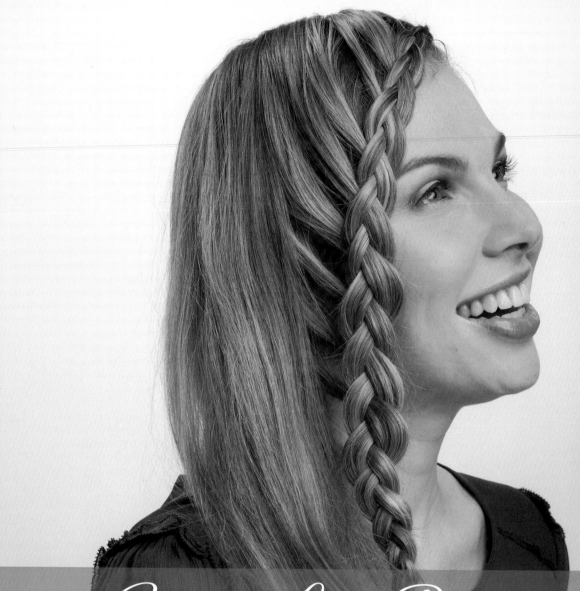

Fringe Lace Braid

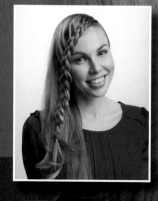

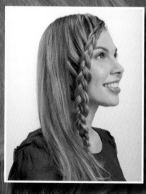

You'll be front and center at every weekend barbecue and festival with the Fringe Lace Braid. Fun and flirty, this super-girly style is a great look to celebrate the spring and summer months. Plus, you'll be able to play all day without worrying about creating a mess of this braid.

Here, we'll learn the lace braiding technique to add in hair for a diagonal, cascading waterfall effect. The lace braid frames the face, while adding a really interesting visual detail from the top and sides. This lace braid combines with a Three-Strand Braid (page 17), making it a pretty easy style. Once you get the hang of it, this braid is essentially effortless. You can also try replacing the Three-Strand Braid by adding the lace effect to a Basic Fishtail or a twist. In general, lace braids work best on straight and wavy hair in order to really highlight the pieces of hair added in while braiding.

TIPS FOR PREPPING

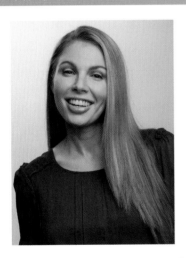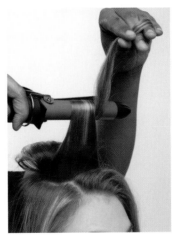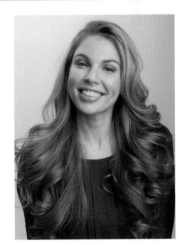

Curled ends add some playfulness to match this flirty braid. Here, the hair was blow-dried with a mousse and gel. Use a round brush to create a slight curl on the ends. With dry hair, use a 1- or 1½-inch curling iron for a similar effect.

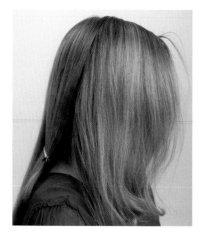

1: Make a diagonal part from the front left corner of the head to behind the right ear. Pin the bottom to keep this section out of the way.

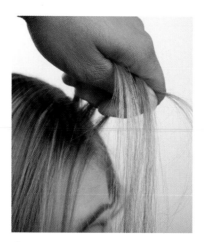

2: Begin at the front left corner of the fringe. Take a small subsection at the part and divide it into 3 strands.

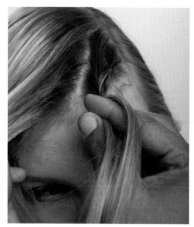

3: Cross the center strand over the right strand. Cross the new center strand over the left strand. Pick up hair to add to the left strand. Cross the left strand under the center strand.

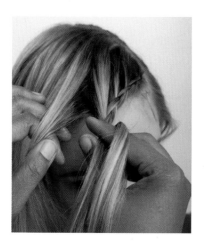

4: Continue this braiding pattern diagonally, continuing to pick up hair only when the left strand crosses under the center strand.

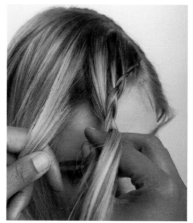

5: Keep the braid at the hairline. As hair is picked up from the left, that hair will extend further.

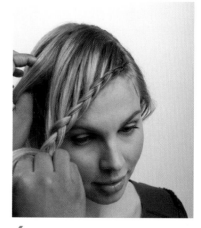

6: Add anti-frizz milk or serum to fingertips while braiding. It is important for this style to be neat. Each time a new subsection of hair is added, run fingers through the hair to remove all tangles.

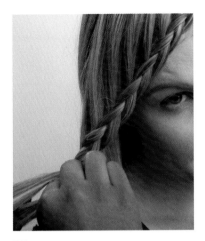

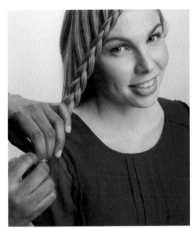

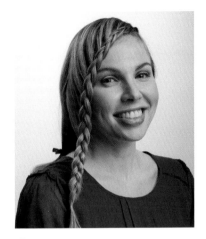

7: While creating this lace braid, leave a little slack to create fullness in later steps. Once all the hair in the front section of the head has been picked up, the lace braid is finished. Transition to Three-Strand Braid.

8: Continue the Three-Strand Braid to the ends of the hair and secure with an elastic band.

TIP: Use a clear plastic band for lighter hair colors.

9: Pancake the braid by gently tugging on each loop. This widens the braid and gives it a more mature look.

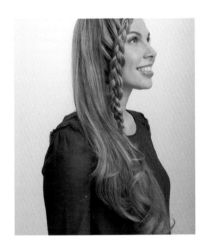

10: Unclip the rest of the hair. Backcomb the ends of the braid to merge it into the loose hair.

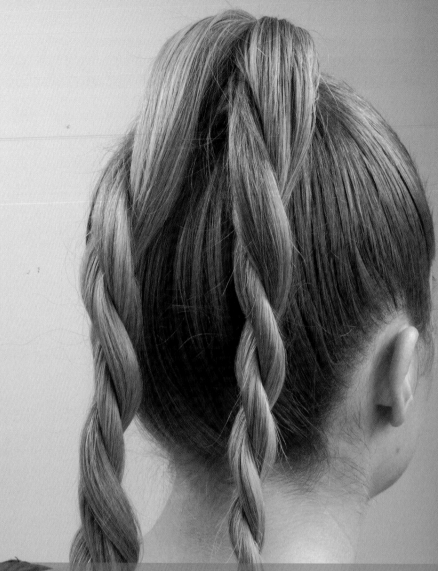

Twisting Techniques

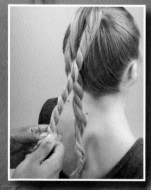

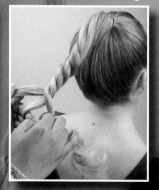

Tornado season comes early with this classic braid technique. Cyclone-inspired twists are actually outside of the traditional "braid" family, but are close style sisters (or cousins, perhaps). Twists will start with either two or three strands, but instead of alternating outer strands, these strands will cross over one another in the same direction each time.

Two- and Three-Strand Twists are my favorites because they're wickedly easy and can be used on any hair type out there. As shown below, you can create a simple pony with two twists for a no-fuss hairstyle. Or spiral a completed twist up into an absolutely perfect messy bun. For that extra chic, textured look, twists look best when you use the pancaking technique. I love incorporating twists into updos, as you'll see in the Five-Braid Updo (page 40) and the Twisted Updo (page 112). Be sure to master these techniques before moving on. Not only is it a great skill to keep in your style toolbox, but you can literally add a twist to your favorite styles by switching out a braid for one of these twists.

Two-Strand Twist

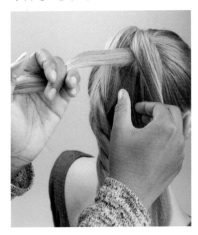
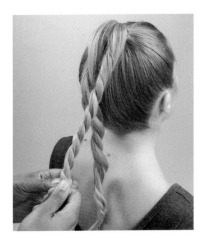
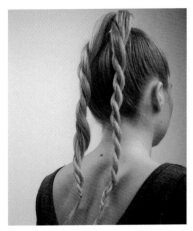

1: Separate hair into two sections. Use a serum to help avoid fly aways.

2: Twist the hair in the same direction either clockwise or counterclockwise. Twist the left strand over the right, and repeat.

3: Continue to twist one strand over the other, since it is only two strands you are simply alternating strands in one direction.

Three-Strand Twist

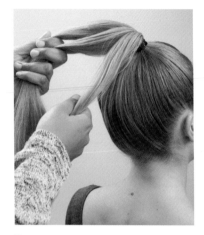

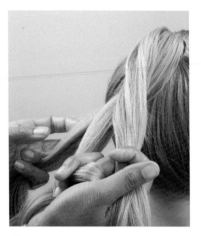

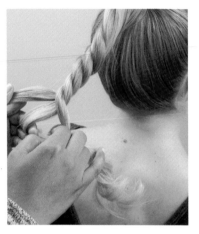

1: Separate the hair into three sections. Use a serum to help you avoid fly aways and keep the twist neat.

2: Twist the center strand over the right, bring the left strand all the way to the right.

3: Cross the new left strand over the right strand, repeat. The rotating option is similar to the rotation of a carousel.

Pancaking

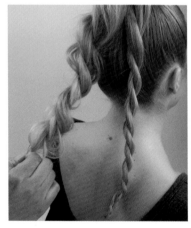

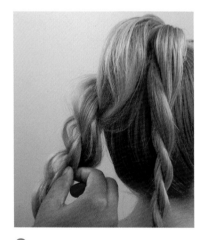

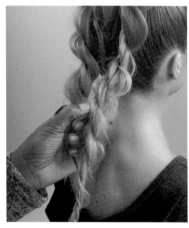

1: Hold the end of one section or strand of the twist. Gently tug on the outside of each loop of the twist.

2: Make sure not to pull the strand out of the twist.

TIP: Focus on one strand at a time.

3: Secure with an elastic band. Pancaking takes practice and finesse, you'll rock it in no time.

Chapter 4
Advanced Braids

When you feel comfortable with simpler braiding techniques and styles, it's time to try out some very sophisticated styles. You'll find the looks in this section, which include updos, crown braids, artistic designs, and others, are more complex. Some feature multiple braids, twists, and layers. But with a little practice and experimentation, the looks in this section offer you a level of sophistication that you can't get with simple braids. These are the looks that are chic enough for a glamorous night on the town and elegant enough to wear on your wedding day.

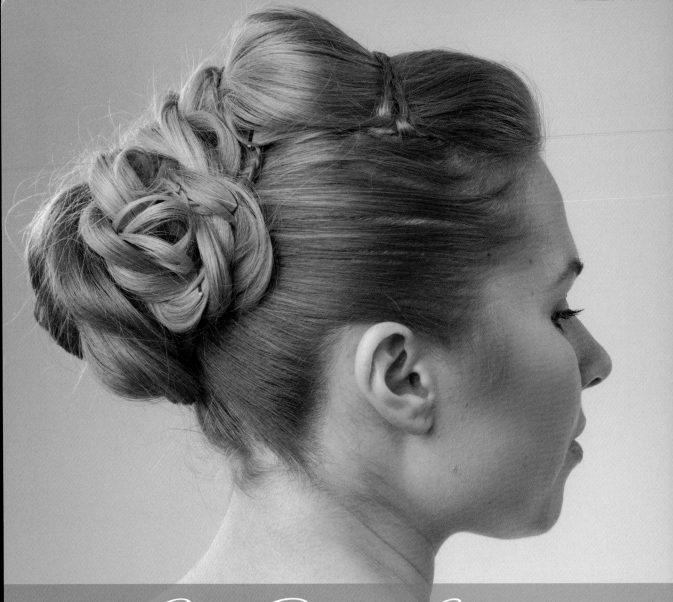

Five-Braid Updo

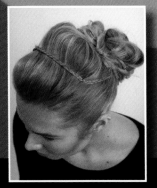
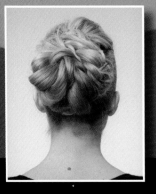
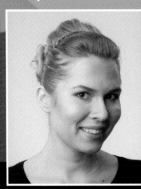

Buckle your seatbelts, this classic-looking updo design has a lot of steps, but it's oh-so-beautiful when you've gotten to the end! The Five-Braid Updo is a bit of a misnomer; technically, it's two basic braids and three braided twists, but regardless, it's perfect for just about anything. It's elegant enough for a wedding and casual enough for a Saturday night. Best of all, because this style is comprised almost entirely of different braids, it's remarkably resilient and will hold for hours.

My favorite thing about this design is that you can really make it your own with a myriad of different options for the back while keeping a clean, polished look from the front and sides. Once you have the braids and twists in place, experiment a little! Layer, bun, and blend the twists in different ways to create the exact look that suits what you're working with.

TIPS FOR PREPPING

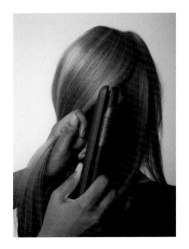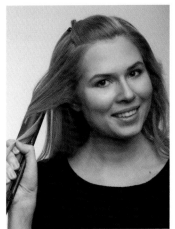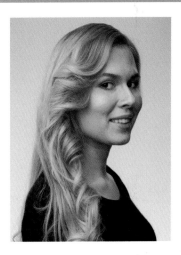

This look definitely works best with straighter hair—either a flat-iron curl, curling iron curls, or just a plain straightening prep. Any updo is going to be able to mask a wide range of textures, but you'll find the small braids and twists required for finishing this particular style a little easier with straighter hair. Highly textured hair can mask the intricacy of the style.

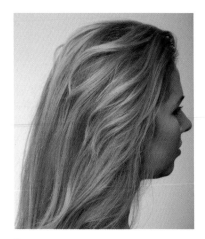

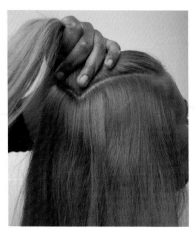

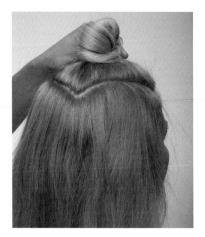

1: Brush the hair straight back, leaving in as much volume as possible while removing any tangles and knots.

2: Isolate the hair from the crown of the head forward, creating a "V" shape at the back of the crown.

3: Twist the section into a small bun and hold it in place using a large bobby pin or clip.

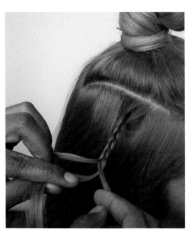

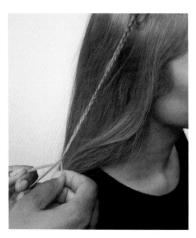

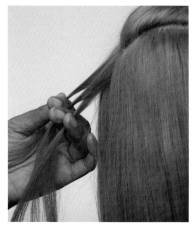

4: Take a small section of hair from the middle-right side of the scalp. Separate the section into three strands and start a Three-Strand Braid (page 17). Leave enough room at the scalp for the braid to move freely.

5: Continue the braid down the hair shaft, tying off the ends with a small, clear elastic band.

6: On the opposite side of the head, at the midpoint of the left side, create a mirror Three-Strand Braid (steps 4 to 5). To ensure a flyaway-free braid, brush out the side before separating the strands.

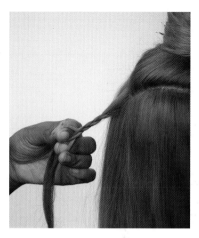

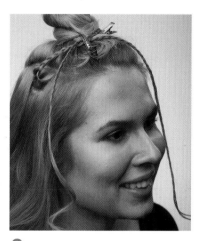

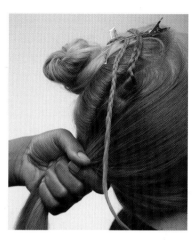

7: Continue braiding the left-side braid down the hair shaft, tying off the ends with another small, clear elastic band.

8: Pin these Three-Strand Braids out of the way for now, as the next steps will be focused on the back of the head. Rest both braids across the top of the head and gently clip.

9: With the bun still held in place along with the two small braids, take hold of all the free hair.

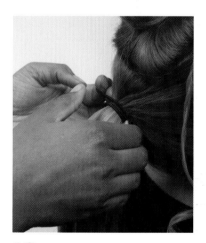

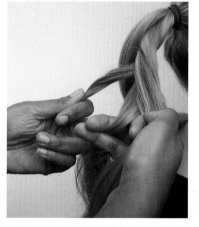

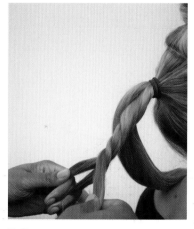

10: Using a thick hair tie, pull the hair back and tie into a tight ponytail at the back of the head.

11: Separate the ponytail into two sections, half on the right and half on the left. Clip the hair on the left out of the way. Take up the right half of the ponytail and begin a Three-Strand Twist (page 38).

12: Unlike a braid, cross strands over one another in the same direction each time to create the twist. Each time a strand crosses over, twist it three times in the reverse direction before crossing the next strand.

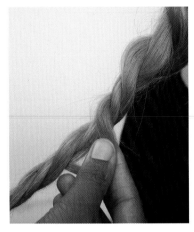

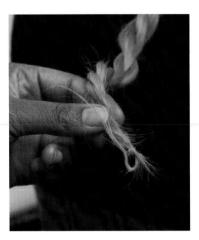

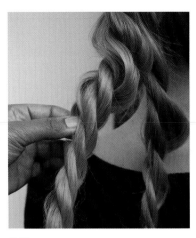

13: Make sure the twist is as full as possible by pulling gently on each strand down the twist.

14: Tie off the first twist with a sturdy, clear elastic. Get as close to the tips as possible, but if the hair is layered or textured, it may need to be a couple inches loose.

15: Repeat steps 12 to 14 on the left side of the ponytail. The twist should be made in the same direction as the one on the right.

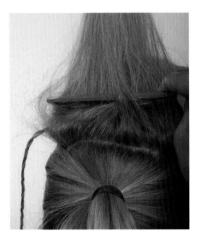

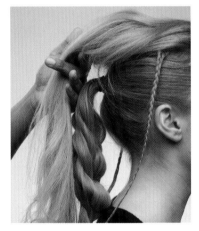

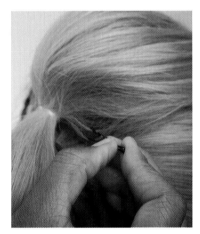

16: Unclip the two small braids and release the bun from the top of the head. Flip hair forward and tease at the base of the scalp with a comb.

17: Flip the hair back and brush the surface. Be careful to keep the teased hair voluminous by brushing gently.

18: Create a high ponytail at the point of the "V" of the crown. Secure with a clear tie. Use bobby pins to keep volume from collapsing.

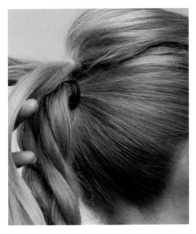

19: Separate the ponytail into three distinct strands directly above the two lower twists.

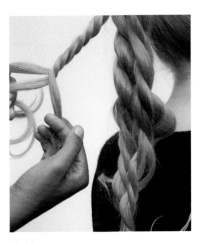

20: Using the three strands, create another Three-Strand Twist. This time, be sure to make the twist a bit tighter than the lower ones.

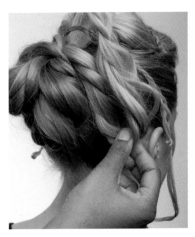

21: Gently lay the small braid from the right side across the top of the head and secure it to the other side with bobby pins.

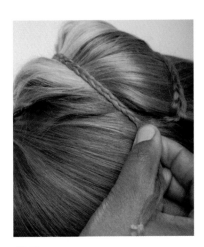

22: Lay left braid across the back of the top ponytail so it pushes up the teased hair and creates a bump at the crown.

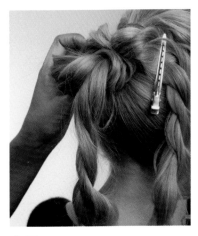

23: Take the left twist from the lower ponytail. Twist it into a bun on the lower left side of the back of the head and secure with bobby pins.

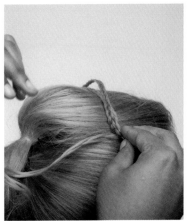

24: Repeat with the lower right twist on the right side. Gently take the top twist from the top ponytail.

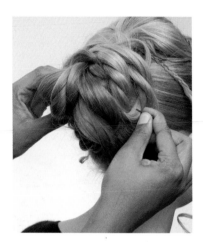 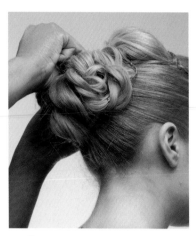 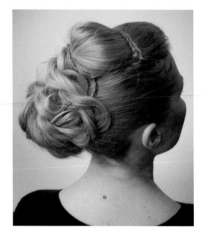

25: Halfway down the top twist, fold the twist on top of itself and gently rest over the two twisted buns.

26: There may be leftover length from the small braids. Incorporate these braids into the design at the back.

27: Be creative when arranging the twists at the back. There are no set rules; pin the strands however looks best.

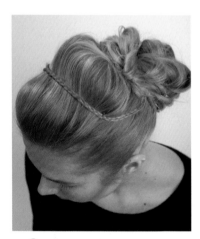

28: Pins are your best friends! Use as many as needed, especially if the style needs to hold for a long while.

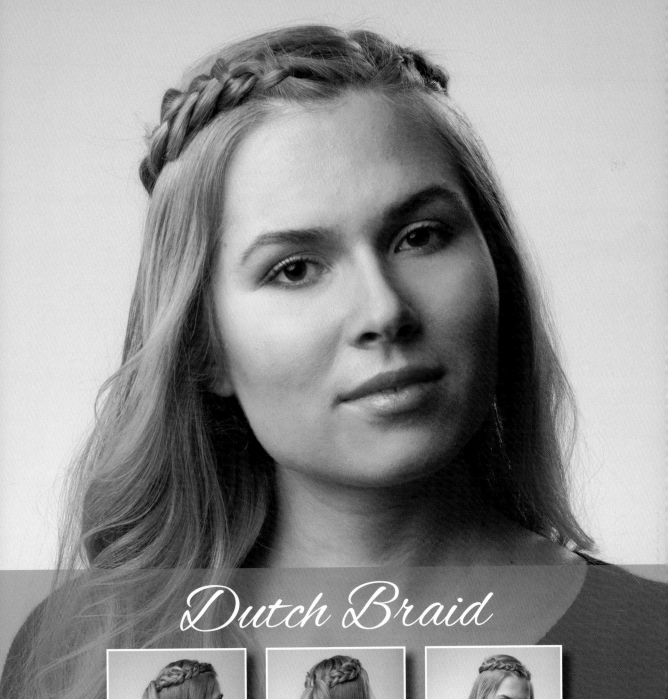

Dutch Braid

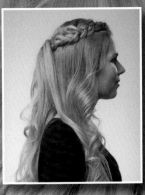
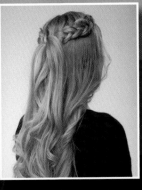
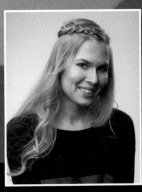

The Dutch Braid is your new best friend. This classic braid is extremely versatile; it acts as a solid base for many of the styles in this book and is a stand-out solo braid as well. You may recognize this braid from its popular style sister: the French Braid. The Dutch Braid works underhand, meaning all strands are crossed underneath one another, while the French Braid works overhand, meaning all strands are crossed on top of one another.

Here, we've styled the Dutch Braid into a partial updo, creating a lovely crown effect. Perfect for any hair type or texture, it's formed by two laced Dutch Braids on either side of the head to form a boho-style headband. The Dutch Braid can be replaced with any of the standard styles: Basic Fishtail (page 20), Knot Braid (page 24), or Three-Strand Twist (page 38). Just be sure to pick up larger sections from the opposite side of the part to keep the crown's shape.

This look can be worn at weekend festivals, outdoor picnics, or whenever you're looking to add a little magic to casual gatherings. Be sure to secure this style with pins and holding spray.

TIPS FOR PREPPING

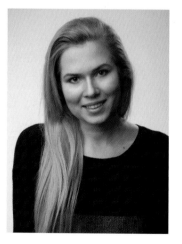 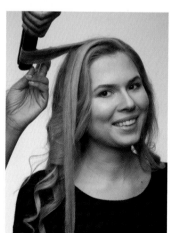 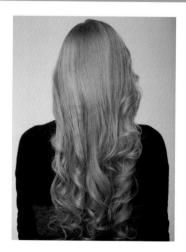

Since this partial updo leaves a good deal of hair loose, flat iron curls added after blow-drying will give the hair a nice wave. Straight hair or tight curls will also look nice with this style.

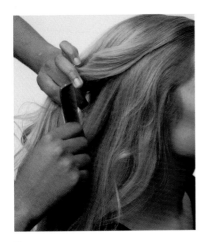

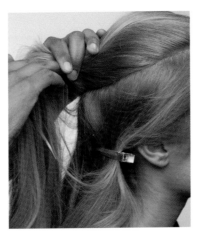

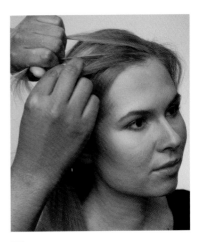

1: Add a deep side part on the left. With a rattail comb, create another part starting from the inside of the right eyebrow.

2: Continue the part toward the center of the head. Create another part from the inside of the left eyebrow to back of head. Parts should meet in the back center to create a deep "V" section.

3: Select a small subsection from the top left corner. Divide hair into three strands. Begin a Dutch Braid.

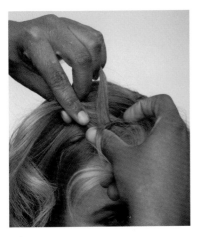

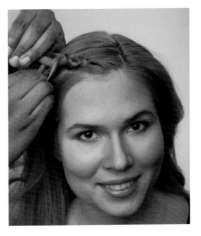

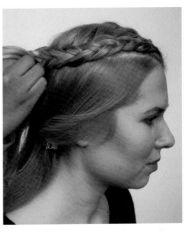

4: Cross the right strand under the center strand. Cross the left strand under the center strand. Pick up hair on either side each time a strand is crossed. Direct Dutch Braid toward the hairline.

5: Repeat. Keep the part close to the right side of the braid; pick up more hair from the left side and less from the right.

6: Braid along the part until reaching the bottom of the "V" at back of head. Secure with an elastic band.

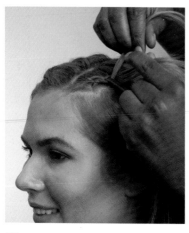

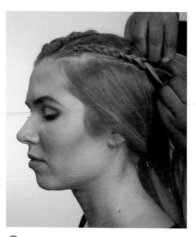

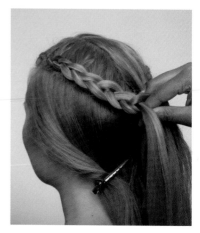

7: Pick up a tiny section from the top right corner of the left section. Divide into three strands and begin a Dutch Braid.

8: Braid alongside the left part, keeping it left of the braid. Pick up larger sections from the right while braiding.

9: Once the laced Dutch Braid reaches the "V" in the back, secure with an elastic band.

TIP: Add a little anti-frizz milk or serum to fingertips while braiding to avoid flyaways.

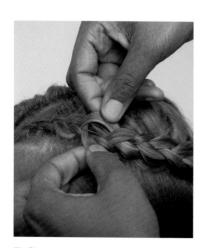

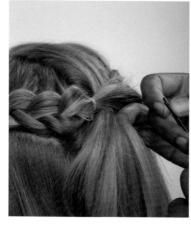

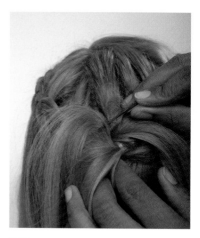

10: For a modern and fashionable look, add width. Use the pancaking technique, gently pulling the outside loops of the braid to loosen and widen.

11: Cross the tail of hair from the left side over the end of the right braid. Bobby pin to secure.

12: Take the tail of the right side under, then over the hair on the left. Bobby pin to secure.

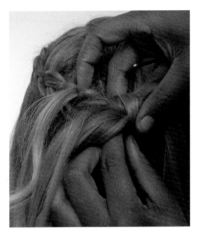

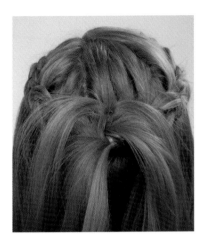

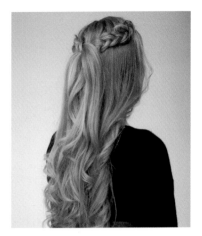

13: Hair is now crossed similar to a Knot Braid (page 24). Cross bobby pins for added security.

14: Pin hair to cover the base of the braids and to hide rubber bands.

15: Allow the rest of the hair to flow loosely. The curled ends of the braids will blend in to the rest of the hair.

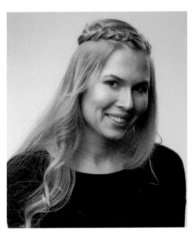

16: Finish with holding spray. Keep this look in mind to spice up boring partial updos!

BACKCOMBING

One of the most useful techniques in styling is backcombing (backbrushing or teasing) the hair. Backcombing can add significant volume to any look and is especially good for fancy updos. Backcombing works by combing the hair against its natural "grain"; each cuticle of hair has small overlapping cells that form scales moving away from the scalp. Backcombing rubs against these scales in the opposite direction, causing the hair to tangle and stack up on top of itself and increase in volume. Here are the simple steps:

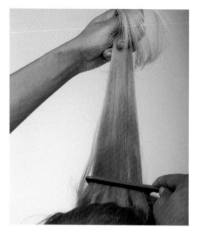

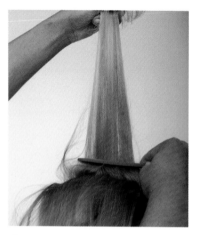

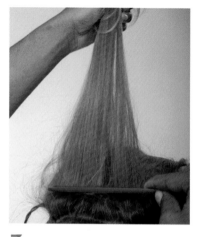

1: Take hold of the 1-inch section of hair you plan to backcomb (normally from the top of the scalp).

2: Slowly run the comb from the middle of the strands, through the section, and down, toward the scalp.

3: Repeat until the hair is visibly teased and more voluminous. Add more 1-inch sections as needed.

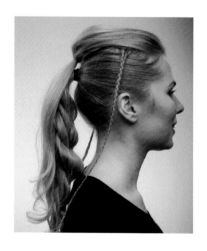

The Results

Lay the backcombed section into the look. Here you can see the increased volume at the crown of the head.

TIP: To remove the backcombed section, gently comb the section starting at the ends and moving toward the roots. Once you reach the roots, the tangles should be loosened or removed.

TIP: While backcombing can add drama to most styles, remember that repeated backcombing can cause significant damage to your hair cuticles if done improperly or too roughly. It's definitely best to save the technique for special occasions, especially if you have long hair to maintain.

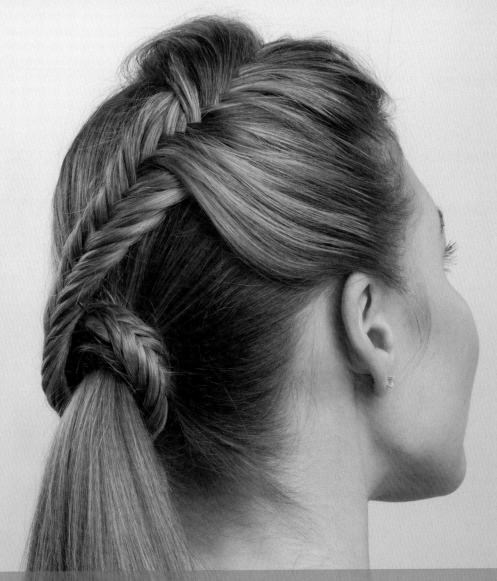

French Fishtail Pony

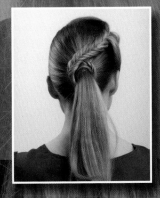
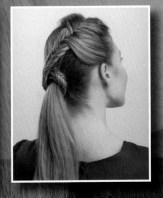
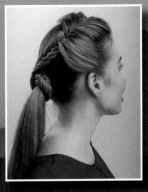

Bonjour mon chéri! In this braid, we'll incorporate aspects of the classic French Braid into the fishtail for a sporty yet detailed braid. This look is perfect for keeping hair out of your face, whether you're hunkering down at the daily grind or backpacking through Europe. The French Fishtail Pony is not only pretty and practical, it's pretty easy to boot! The detail in the fishtail makes this look like a complicated braid, but it's only a touch different from the Basic Fishtail. This look works best on wavy and straight hair types—the detail really pops against straighter hair.

If you're looking to take this look a few steps further, check out variation of the style on page 58 and page 61. You can also try out a Dutch Braid, Three-Strand Braid, or Knot Braid page 24) in the place of the French Fishtail, as long as you pick up hair as you go along for the "French effect." You'll be touring in style with this look; it won't fall apart until you're ready to say *au revoir* for the night.

TIPS FOR PREPPING

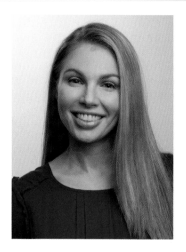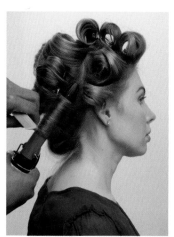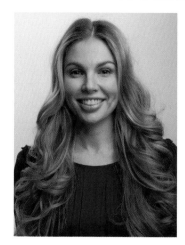

Loose curls were chosen for this style to help easily mold the braid. Hair was blow-dried with mousse and a thermal setting spray. Curls were added with a 1-inch tourmaline curling iron. Blow-drying or curling can be chosen if time is of the essence.

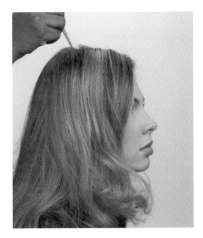

1: Create a side part. For the best look, align the part at the arch of the eyebrow.

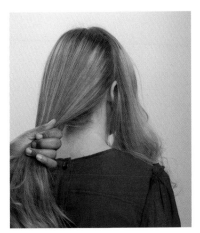

2: Take the part back 3 inches. Extend the part horizontally to the back of the left ear, creating an L-shaped section.

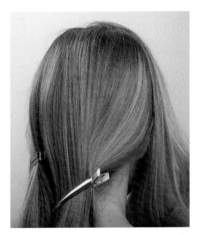

3: Once the L-shaped crown section has been created, use duckbill clips to separate each section. Add a small amount of hair spray or anti-frizz serum to smooth flyaways.

TIP: Duckbill clips are long, curved clips that contour to the shape of the head. They're ideal for holding hair out of the way during styling.

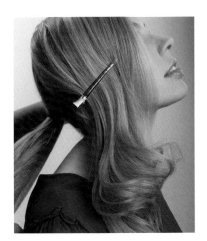

4: Gather a low ponytail in the back section. Tilt head back for smoother ponytails. Secure with an elastic hair tie.

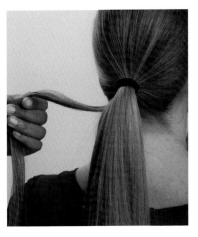

5: Take a small piece of hair from the ponytail. Use anti-frizz serum to smooth the small piece.

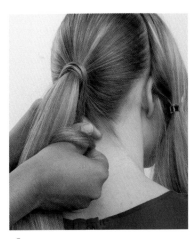

6: Carefully wrap hair around the base of the ponytail at least two times. Stop the wrap just under the ponytail.

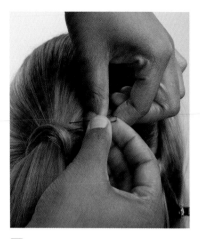

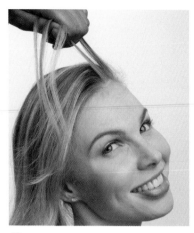

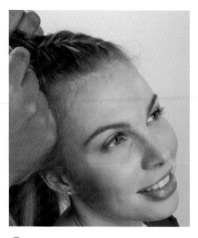

7: Using a small colored hair pin, secure the small piece of hair from underneath the pony. Make sure the elastic band is completely covered by the pinned hair for a more finished look.

8: On the crown section, you will begin a French fishtail braid. Take a small section and divide into 2 strands.

9: Begin the fishtail. Take hair from behind the right strand, cross that hair over the right strand and add it to left. Repeat on left strand.

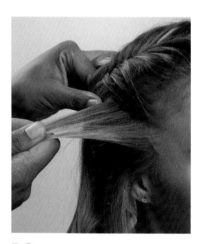

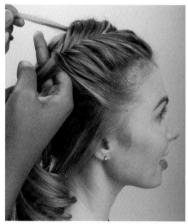

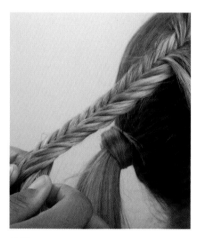

10: Each time hair from behind is crossed over and added to the opposite strand, pick up and add hair from the scalp into the other side, like a French Braid.

11: Direct the French fishtail braid around the head, toward the back of the right ear. Don't braid super-tight here—leave some space between the braid and the scalp. This will help direct the braid.

12: After the hair from the top section has been picked up by the French fishtail, transition to a Basic Fishtail by taking hair from the back of the right section over and around the right strand and adding it to the left section. Repeat this on the left side.

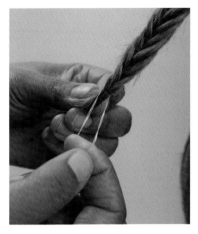

13: Once the fishtail reaches the ends, secure with an elastic band.

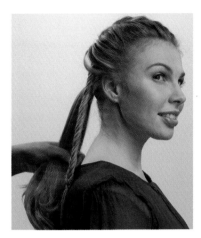

14: Make sure that there is some slack at the base of the braid so it can be moved easily.

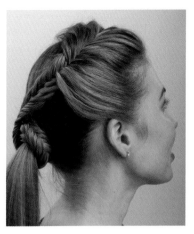

15: Wrap the fishtail around the base of the ponytail. Pin the fishtail braid around the base.

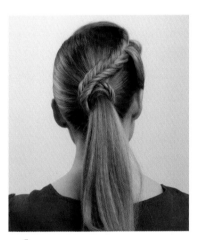

16: If there are any gaps between the fishtail and the ponytail base, use hair pins to close the gap.

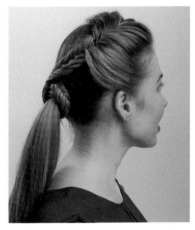

17: Brush out the ponytail gently. Finish the style with a spray serum and holding spray.

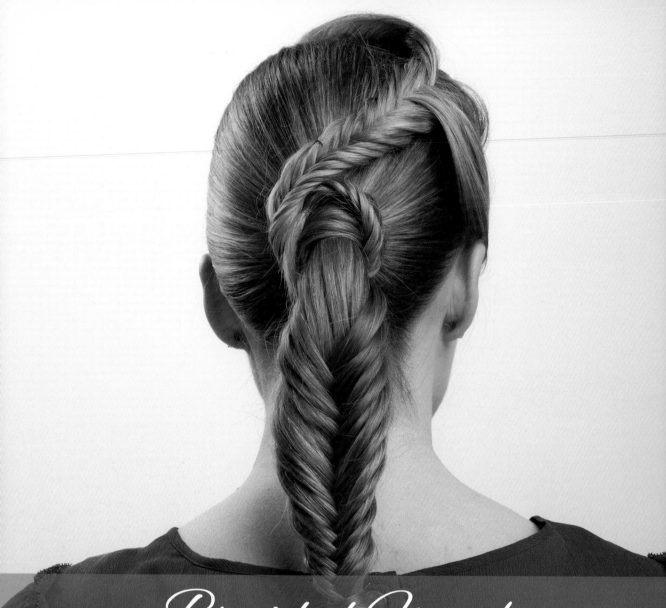

Braided French Fishtail Pony

(Variation)

By now you've mastered the French Fishtail, so this should be an easy next step. An added French fishtail creates a compelling extension of the style from the crown to ends. This adds a little more security to the hair, not to mention tons of extra detail. With hair out of the way, this look is good for work, hanging out with friends, or even playing a sport.

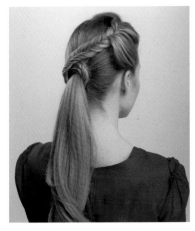

1: Start with the completed French Fishtail Pony from page 53.

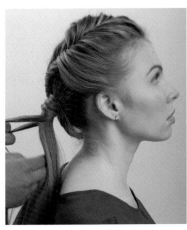

2: Loosen the fishtail braid pinned around the base of the ponytail. Take up a small section from the ponytail base.

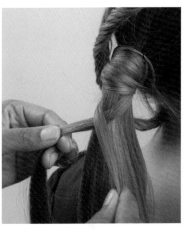

3: Divide the section into two. Begin a fishtail by crossing the right over the left and the left over the right.

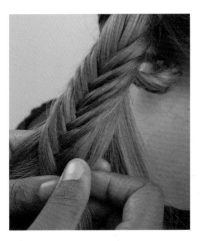

4: Keep braiding in hair from the back of the pony to either side (alternating left over right and then right over left).

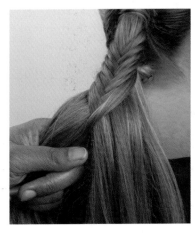

5: Continue braiding until all hair in the ponytail has been picked up. There should only be two strands.

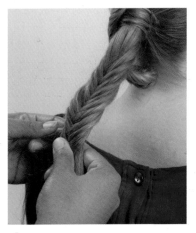

6: Holding each side firmly while braiding, continue the fishtail braid until you are a few inches from the ends.

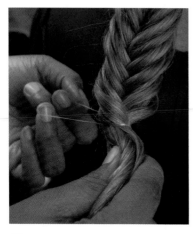

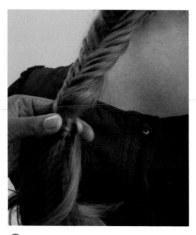

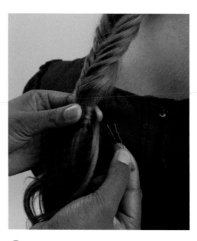

7: Secure the braid with an elastic band. Leaving a few inches at the ends offers a flirty look.

8: Take a tiny subsection of hair from the bottom of the braid and wrap it around the elastic.

9: Using a small hair-colored bobby or hair pin, secure the section so it hides the elastic for a finished look.

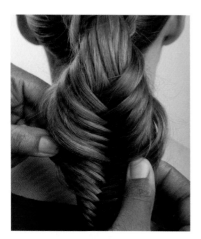

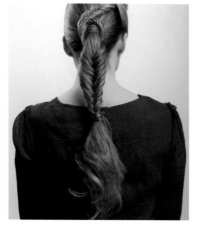

10: Loosen the braid to add fullness. Wrap the top fishtail braid back around the base of the ponytail and pin.

11: Backcomb the bottom of the braid to add body to the curls. Finish with a holding spray.

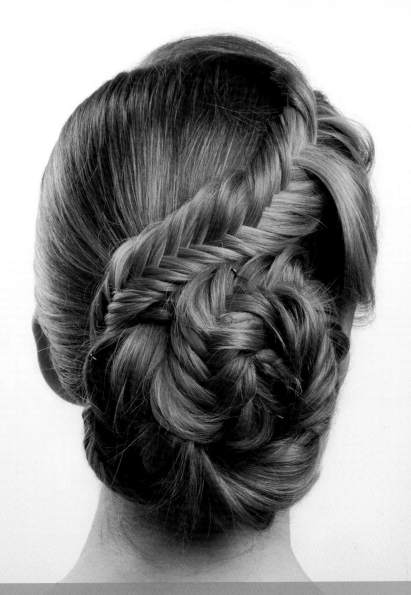

French Fishtail Updo

(Variation)

Embody elegance with this final variation of the French Fishtail Pony. A few small changes completely transform the feel of this style, going from a sporty ponytail to a black-tie updo. Believe it or not, this look is surprisingly easy. It's all about your bobby pin skills here; as long as you can place a pin, you'll be turning heads at every wedding, prom, or formal occasion.

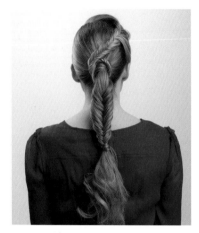

1: Start with the completed French Fishtail Pony (page 53). We'll turn this fun style into an elegant updo.

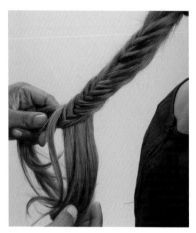

2: Unwrap the top fishtail braid from the base of the ponytail. Remove elastic from the bottom of the ponytail fishtail.

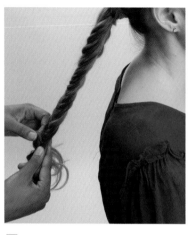

3: Continue the fishtail braid down to the ends. Cross a right strand over and into the left, the left over into the right.

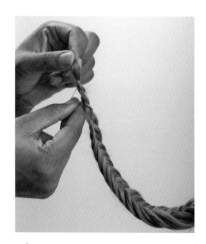

4: Secure with a hair-colored elastic band.

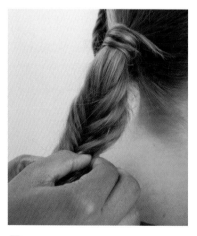

5: Widen the braid using the pancaking technique (page 38).

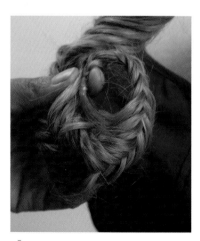

6: Starting with the end of the braid, begin rolling the fishtail toward the top of the ponytail.

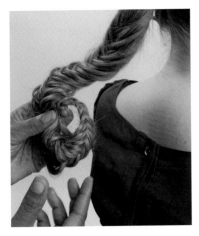

7: Since the fishtail is flat, roll the braid so the braid stays flat and wide, rather than on its side.

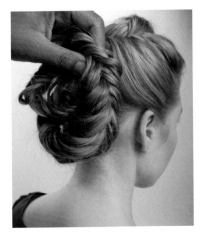

8: Roll the fishtail braid up to the scalp. Widen the shape of the rolled-up braid to resemble a flower.

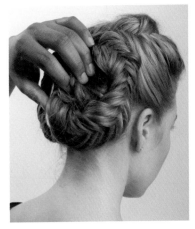

9: Alternate between long bobby pins and hair pins to secure the flower. Make sure the pins match the hair color.

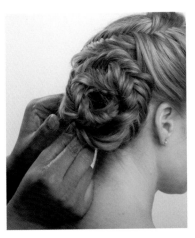

10: Weave pins in and out of the braid and hair at the scalp. Cross pins for extra security. This braid is heavy and needs extra support to last all evening.

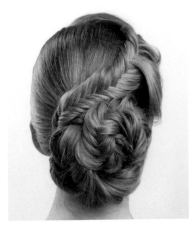

11: Pin the top fishtail braid around the left side of the flower. For extra detail, pin the fishtail stitches directly into the flower.

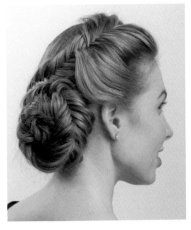

12: This creates a gorgeous side updo!

TIP: Side updos look best for formal events and photos.

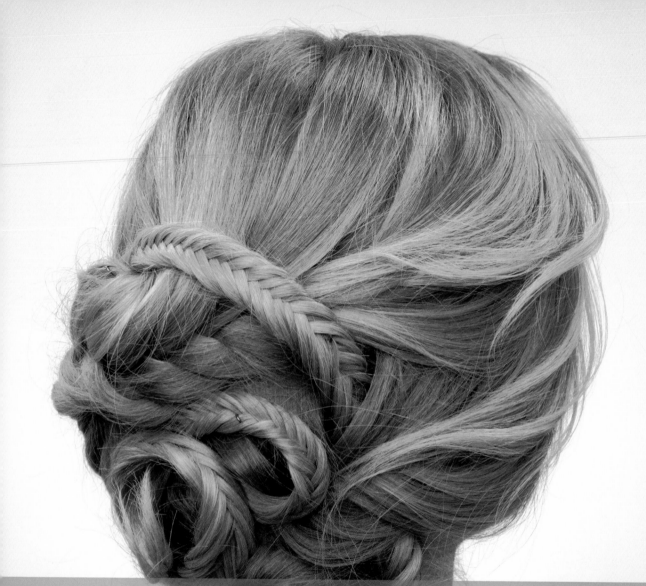

The Triple Mermaid Updo

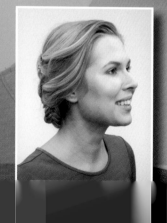
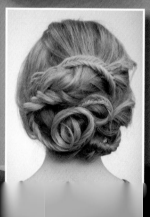
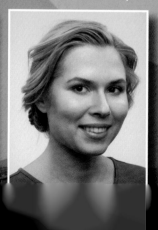

Few have ever caught a glimpse of the mermaid, a rare sighting from myth and legend. But you can make this an everyday encounter with this splashy, special occasion updo. With not one, not two, but three fishtails that intertwine, this ocean-inspired look will leave your fellow partygoers feeling like they've just seen something magical.

And they would have! The Triple Mermaid Updo does have a bit of magic to it. This is a more complicated style; it definitely requires a mastery of the Basic Fishtail (page 20), along with the French Fishtail Pony (page 53) and Fringe Lace Braid (page 32) techniques. We'll be combining all three in this look and then weaving them together in a pattern that resembles rolling waves. But don't actually get this one wet! If you stay ashore and secure it with pins, this updo will stay in all night.

If fishtails are a little too advanced, try out this style with Dutch Braids and Three-Strand Braids to get a similar look. I recommend this look on straightened or wavy hair. Using a flat iron can help the detail in the fishtail braids stand out more, especially when it comes to the lace fishtails.

TIPS FOR PREPPING

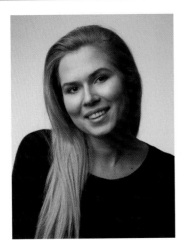 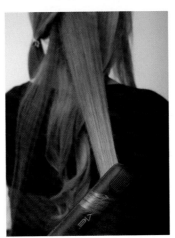 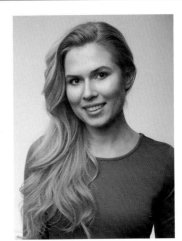

Try this look on flat-ironed, roller-set, or naturally straight hair. Personally, I love the way this style looks on straight and wavy hair. With straighter hair, the details really pop.

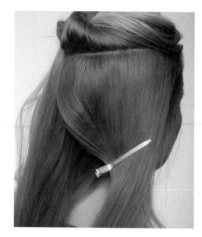

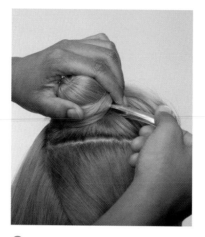

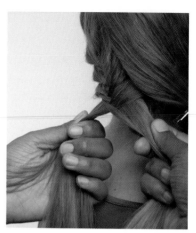

1: Create a diagonal part from the arch of the left brow, behind the head, toward the back of the right ear. Part hair from the arch of the right brow toward the center of the head. Stop when you reach the first part, creating a triangle.

2: Clip the triangular section on top of the head into a bun. Clip away remaining hair on the right side.

TIP: Since this style is all about detail, add a defrizz milk to aid in braiding.

3: Begin a French Fishtail Pony (page 53). Direct the French fishtail braid diagonally, picking up small sections of hair on each side, until you reach the nape of the neck.

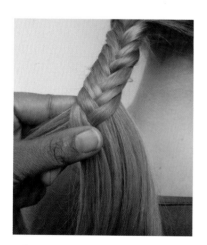

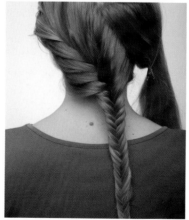

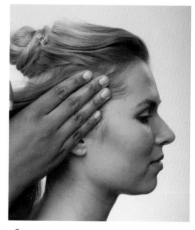

4: At the nape of the neck, begin a Basic Fishtail. Choose hair from the back of the right strand, cross over the right strand, and add it to the left. Repeat.

5: Continue to the ends of the hair. Taking smaller sections when creating the fishtail braid will add extra detail. Secure the bottom of the braid with an elastic band.

6: Smooth the hairline on the right side with a light gel and direct hair away from the face.

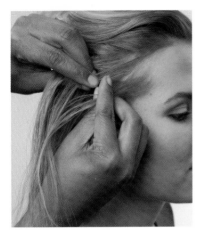

7: Starting from the top corner, take up a small subsection and divide into two strands.

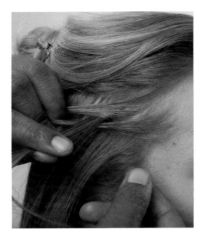

8: Begin a French fishtail braid, adding small sections of hair to the left and right sides until there is no longer hair to pick up from the back of the scalp.

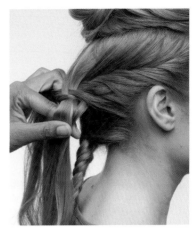

9: Once you reach the back of the head, begin a Basic Fishtail.

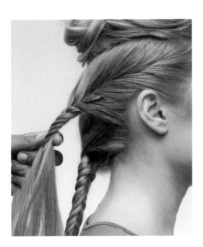

10: When fishtail braiding here, take care to use tiny subsections from the back of the strands for added elegance and detail. Continue the fishtail braid to the end of the hair and secure with an elastic band.

TIP: Use elastic bands similar to hair color. I'm using clear here for a chic look.

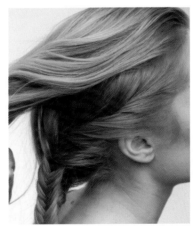

11: Loosely gather hair from the top section in one hand and separate into two strands.

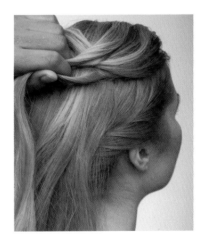

12: Begin a French fishtail braid until reaching the back of the head. Then, transition to a Basic Fishtail.

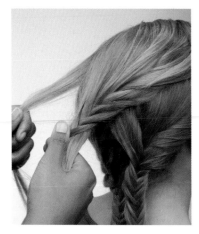

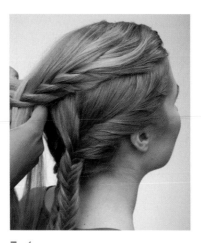

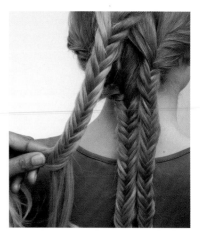

13: Direct the braid to the center of the head by stretching hair form the left side toward the right.

14: To make the fishtail braid look fuller, twist each strand before crossing it into its new section.

15: Continue the fishtail braid down the length of hair and secure ends with an elastic band.

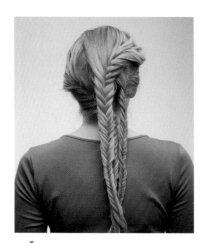

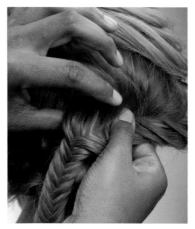

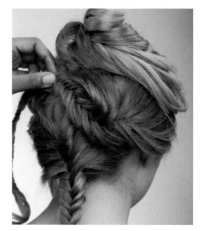

16: Now that all of the braids are complete and secure, it's time to have some styling fun!

17: Clip the top section out of the way. Gently loosen the loops of the braid on the right side.

18: Bobby pin the right braid over the diagonal parting. This also serves as the base of the style.

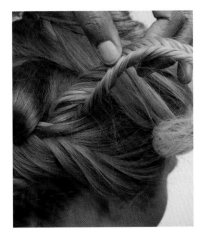

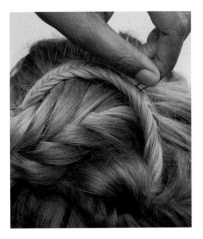

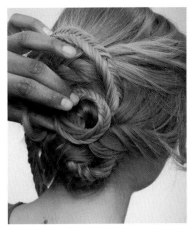

19: Snake the bottom braid under and through the space between the right braid and scalp. This looks trickier than it is!

20: Bring down the top braid. Direct the braid to the left, wrap around toward the nape of the neck, and bobby pin into place. Roll loose ends into loops and pin anywhere.

21: Feel free to twist loose ends and pin them into the style wherever you wish. Get creative with it!

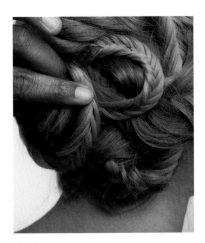

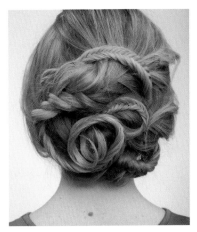

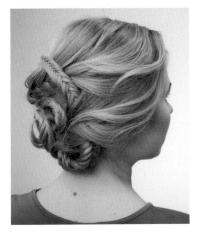

22: Hair pins are crucial for this style. Use hair-colored hair pins throughout the braids to discreetly hold this style in place.

23: Pin the end of a fishtail braid over the top fishtail braid. This frames the style, adding texture and detail.

24: This elegant style is completely customizable. Just make sure to cover any gaps in the style with a braid.

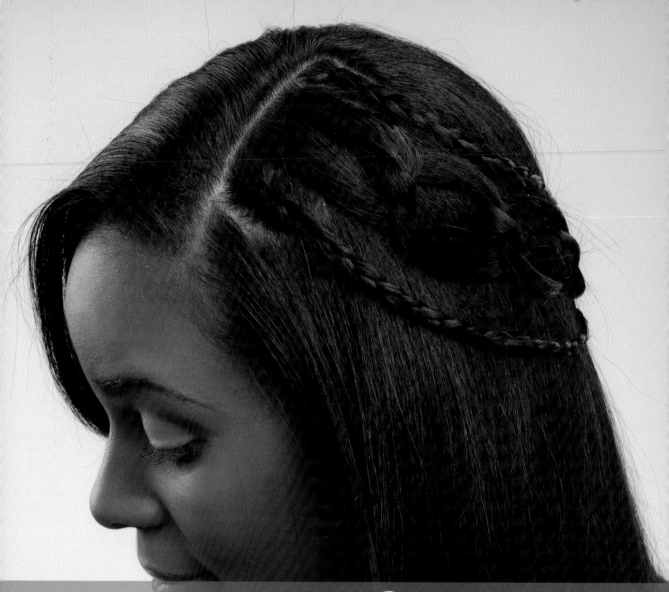

Draped Knot Braid

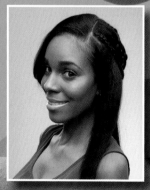
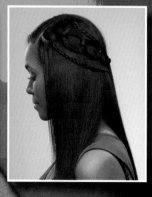
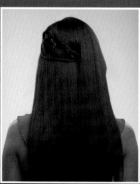

Don't underestimate this simple half-up style. Easy to create, this ultimate day-to-night look is an instant eye-catcher and extremely versatile, whether you're booked for an early morning brunch or a night out with the girls. The cascading detail of the Draped Knot Braid adds a touch of delicate intrigue to normally straight or flat-ironed hair. I definitely recommend that the hair be straightened for this look; I love the way the knot braid stands out against bone-straight locks.

This style starts with two basic Three-Strand Braids, which eventually frame the intricate-looking knot braid in the middle. The technique here is actually one you've already known for years—the knot braid is exactly the same as the first in tying your shoes, so simple a preschooler can do it! If you're looking for more of a challenge, change up this style by switching out the knot braid with a fishtail braid. Or, change the Three-Strand Braids to Three-Strand Twists. Once pinned back, you can guarantee that these braids will make it all day, or all night.

TIPS FOR PREPPING

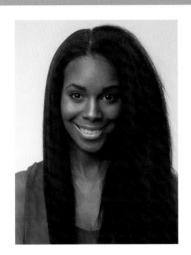 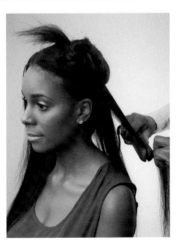 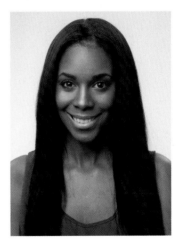

For this super-straight base style, blow-dry hair straight with mousse and a styling brush, then flat iron extra straight with a thermal setting spray and spray serum. If hair is naturally straight, simply add spray shine.

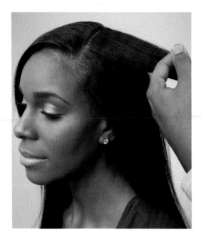

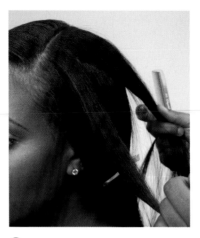

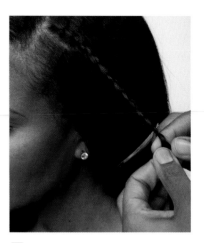

1: Create a deep side part on the left side of the head.

2: Create a rectangle section of hair that starts 1 inch back from the front hairline; it should be 4 inches wide and 1 inch deep. Divide into three, and braid.

3: In the first section, create a Dutch Braid (page 47) and end with a Three-Strand Braid (page 17). Secure with a rubber band.

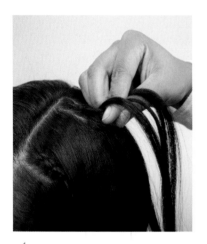

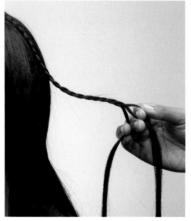

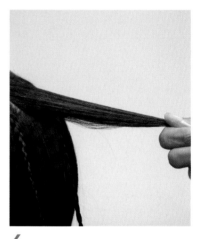

4: Repeat step 3 with the last section. When Dutch braiding this section, make sure not to pick up hair from the middle section. Direct the Dutch Braid down to make styling easier.

TIP: Apply a little serum or anti-frizz milk to fingertips while braiding to minimize frizz and create a more polished style.

5: End the Dutch Braid with a Three-Strand Braid. Secure with a rubber band.

TIP: A clear plastic band can also be used.

6: Take the middle section and divide it into two equal strands. Wrap one strand over, then under, and pull through the loop to create the first knot. It's like the first step of tying a shoe.

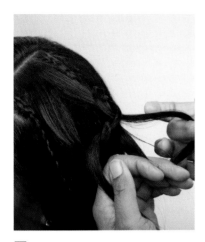

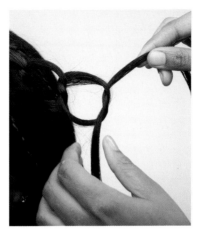

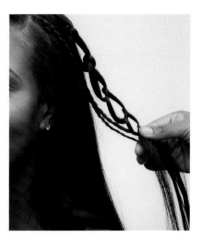

7: Move an inch farther down the strand and begin another knot. It's all about leaving extra space here. The space between the knots creates a really awesome detail.

8: Continue down the hair shaft and create more knots, slipping the back strand over the front strand. This is where the pattern starts to really stand out.

9: Once there are at least three complete knots in the braid, pick up the two outside braids. Hold all three braids between pointer and thumb.

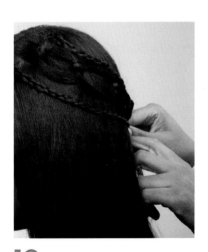

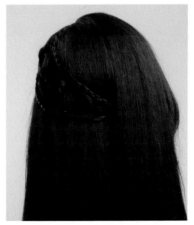

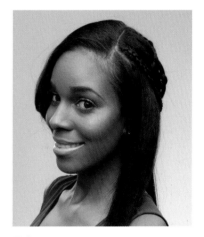

10: Bobby pin all three braids behind the right ear.

TIP: Cross bobby pins for added security.

11: Allow hair from the right side of the head to fall over the pins to hide the crossed bobby pins.

12: Finish the style with a spray shine and a holding spray.

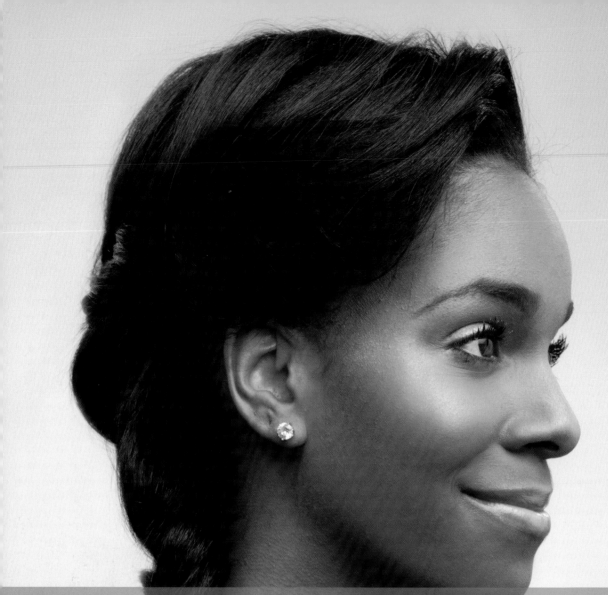

The Fairy Princess

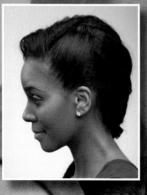 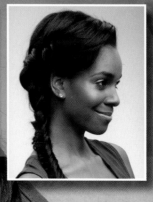 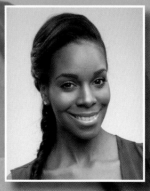

Enchant onlookers with the sleek elegance of this fabulous side braid. You should try this magical look once you've mastered the basics of the fishtail. The Fairy Princess is all about combining the fishtail with the art of sectioning. Have your rattail comb and duckbill clips handy—you'll be making a series of sections, all of which come together to create one extremely detailed, textured, and voluminous fishtail. To make sure all your hard work doesn't go unnoticed, try this look on bone-straight hair. As with most fishtail styles, straighter hair creates much more detail in the final product. If your hair is shorter, try twisting or tucking the fishtail braid into the bottom of the style. Instead of the long side braid, you'll end up with an even more sophisticated updo.

You will be the belle of the ball at fancy dinners and formal events when you sweep in with this style. Don't be afraid to let go—this look will last through a night of dinner and dancing.

TIPS FOR PREPPING

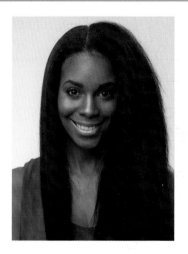 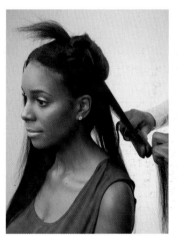 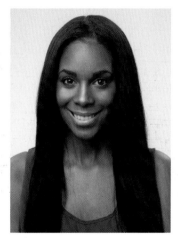

Smooth, flat-ironed, super-straight hair makes the details in this fishtail really pop. If hair is naturally straight or wavy, that works too. This model's hair was blow-dried with a paddle brush, serum, and thermal setting spray. A 1-inch flat iron was used to straighten.

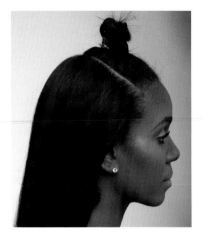

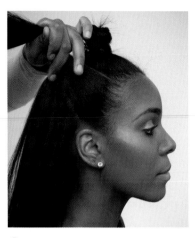

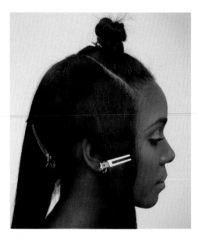

1: Part from the arch of each eyebrow back. Meet parts to create a "V" shaped section at the crown. Clip hair out of way.

2: Starting above the ear on the right side, part upward to meet the corner of the "V" shape. This creates a new "V" section.

3: Pin the side "V" section out of the way.

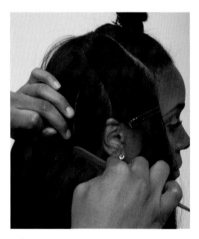

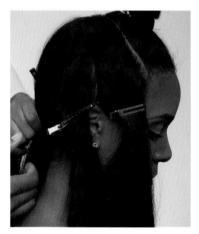

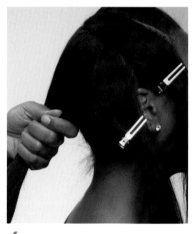

4: Starting 2 inches above the ear, part down and behind from the side section to the nape of the neck.

5: Use a duckbill clip to move hair out of the way. Repeat sectioning steps 2 to 4 on the left side.

6: Next, gather unsectioned hair in the center of the head.

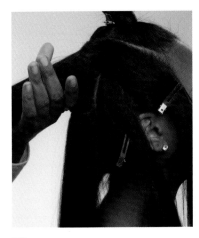

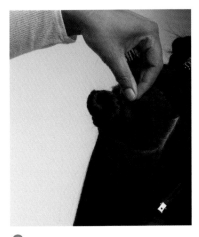

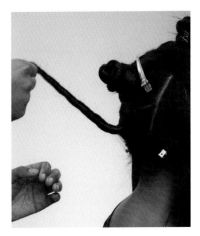

7: Divide this large section horizontally, creating two equal sections.

8: Secure the top section of hair out of the way with a duckbill clip.

9: With the bottom section, twist hair from root to end.

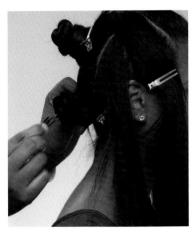

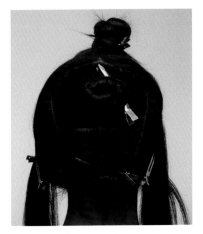

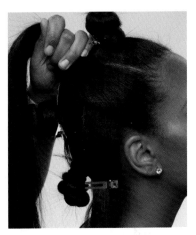

10: Twist hair down to scalp until it makes a cinnamon roll shape. Secure with duckbill clip.

11: At this point, the back of the head will have 7 sections. By the end, there will be a total of 9.

12: Release upper side sections on both sides. Apply hair gel or paste to brush hair smoothly from the hairline. Important: This section must be very neat!

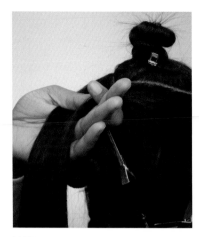

13: Gather both sections from each side into a center ponytail. Use a hair-colored elastic band to secure.

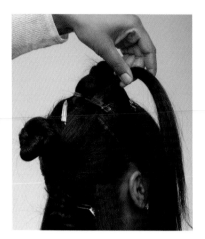

14: Divide the lower side sections on each side in half. Brush the new upper sections into a ponytail at the center. Secure with an elastic band.

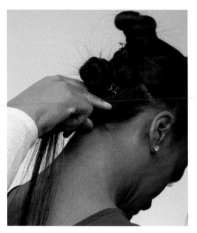

15: Brush the two remaining side sections and gather them into a ponytail at the nape of neck, under the bottom bun. Pull the tail of the pony to tighten.

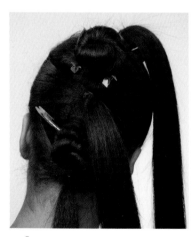

16: This is the back of the head with fully sectioned hair and all ponytails in place.

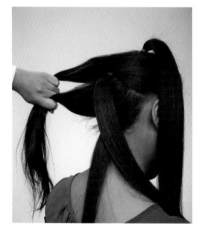

17: Remove all of the clipped, twisted center buns. Let hair hang straight.

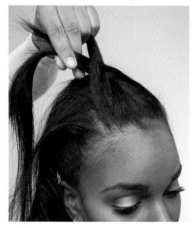

18: Begin a French fishtail at the top left corner of the crown. Direct the braid toward the right side.

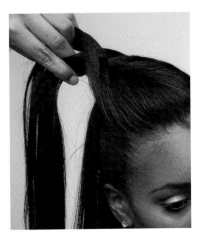

19: Loosely fishtail braid, adding in medium pieces of hair from the scalp on either side.

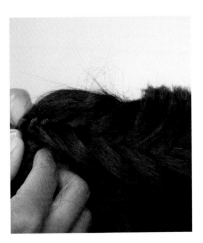

20: At the end of the scalp section, push the hair forward. Gently pull pieces closest to hairline to create volume.

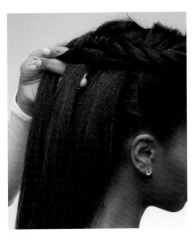

21: The French fishtail is on an angle. Begin adding hair from the uppermost ponytail into the fishtail.

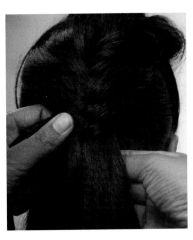

22: As pieces are added in, straighten the braid down the center of the head. Continue the fishtail, adding hair in from the middle section as well.

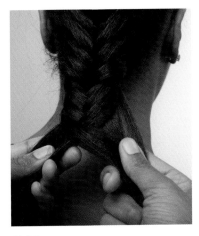

23: Continue the French fishtail braid, picking up the open sections and small ponytails once the braid reaches that area. Once away from the scalp and all sections are picked up, continue with a Basic Fishtail braid.

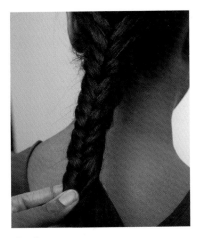

24: Since there is no additional hair to pick up, continue with the Basic Fishtail to the ends. Secure with an elastic band.

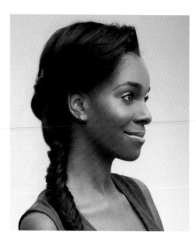 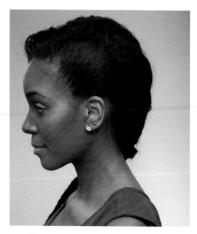

25: Use the pancaking method to widen the braid and add more volume and texture. It also adds a fashionable look.

26: Make sure the hairline is smooth. Add an extra personal touch with ornaments like flowers or fun clips!

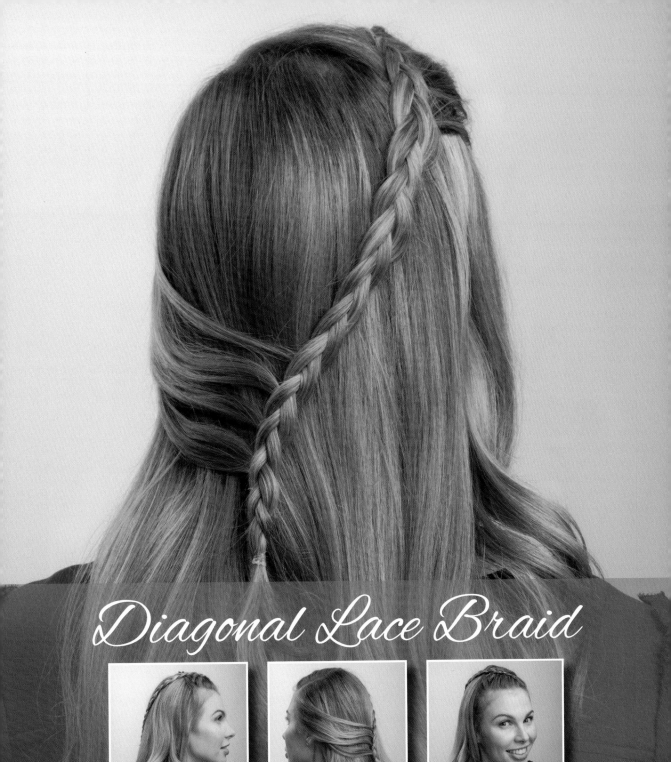

Diagonal Lace Braid

A delicate twist on the Fringe Lace Braid (page 32), this whimsical partial updo is a combination of three different styles. A Dutch Braid (page 47) in front frames the face and keeps those bangs in check, a Three-Strand Braid secures it in place, and a lace braid in the back adds an ethereal touch that makes this a perfect indie style. The lace braid is more advanced, but the end result is well worth it for this awesome fairy-tale look. Fortunately, once you master the lace braid, you can add this boho detail to any other braiding technique, enhancing even the Basic Fishtail, French Braid, and Three-Strand Twist. This style is suited for finer hair and works best with medium- to long-length hair.

Perfect for any occasion, you'll turn heads whether you're making an appearance at a family event or rocking out at a weekend musical festival. Better yet, feel free to dance your heart out; you can have fun until the sun comes up without worrying about this braid coming undone.

TIPS FOR PREPPING

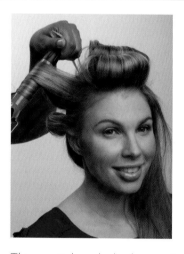 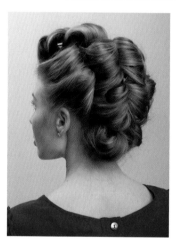 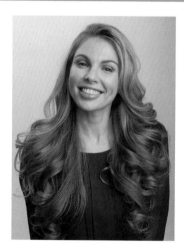

This partial updo looks great with straight hair, but adding some waves into the mix creates an extra detail that offsets the style well. Using a 1-inch curling iron, curl and pin the hair into place to cool. This gives hair a little bounce and lovely waves.

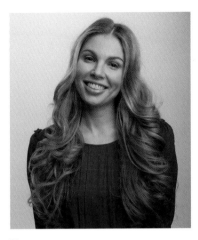

1: Brush through the 1-inch curls and make sure hair is free of tangles.

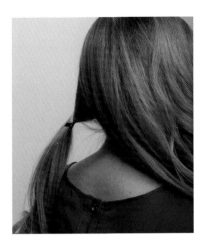

2: Create an L-shaped part from the outer edge of the left eyebrow to behind the right ear. Secure with a duckbill clip.

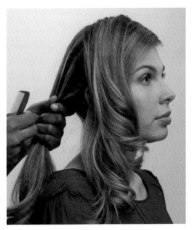

3: Part hair horizontally from the top of the crown to behind the right ear. Secure with a duckbill clip.

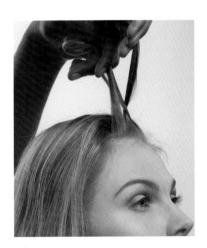

4: Pick up a small section of hair in the top left corner. Divide it into three strands and begin a Dutch Braid (page 47).

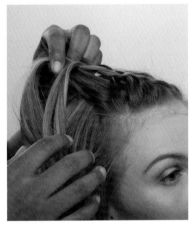

5: Cross the right strand under the center. Cross the left strand under the center. Repeat. Direct diagonally from the left toward the right.

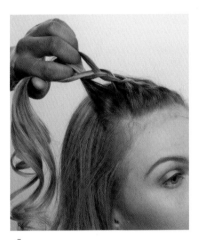

6: While braiding, direct the Dutch Braid toward the right ear. Continue the braid until the top bangs have been picked up. This creates a diagonal effect.

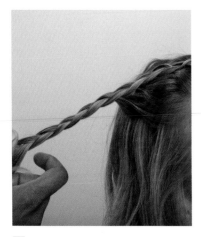

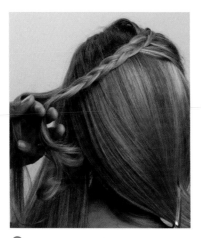

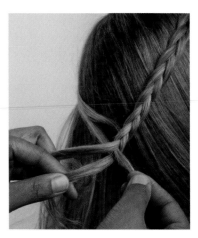

7: Once the Dutch Braid is completed on the top of head, continue down the hair shaft with a Three-Strand Braid (page 17). This braid will be the main focus of the style.

8: Direct the Three-Strand Braid toward the left side of the head where the hair was sectioned off in step 1. This section will be added into the style to create the lace braid.

9: Lace the braid by adding hair from the left side section to the strand currently on the left side of braid.

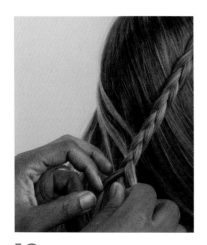

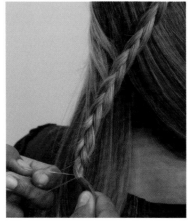

10: Continue the braid, adding hair from the left section only to the strand currently on the left side of the braid.

11: Once all of the hair in the left section has been laced in, complete with a Three-Strand Braid. Secure with a clear elastic band. Let the ends hang free and blend into the rest of the hair.

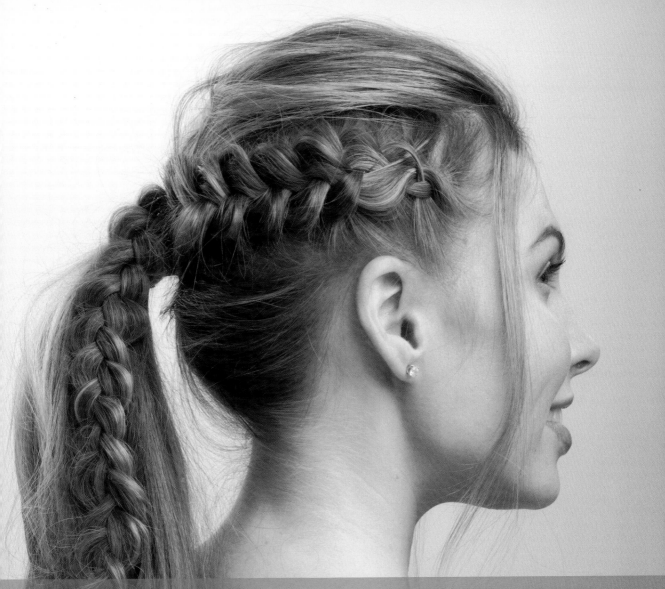

Side Braid Pony

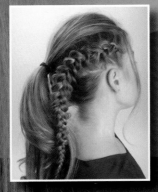
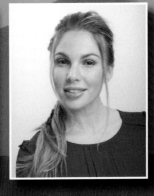

This practical pony is a great time-saver, perfect for those days when you've slept through the alarm and woken up with serious bedhead. The Side Braid Pony works really well with day-old hair. If you've still got some leftover curls from the night before, try giving this style a whirl. You'll be able to use any partial waves you might still have intact, but also totally transform your entire look. No one will notice that you skipped the chore of washing and drying when you meet up the next morning!

Even if you don't have second-day waves, this looks awesome with a lot of hair types: straight, wavy, or slightly curled. This is a super-easy style that braiders of any level can try out as soon as they've mastered the basic Dutch Braid (page 47). For variations on this look, opt for a different type of braid, like the fishtail. Or, you can create the same look by twisting the pony into a bun or simply letting the hair hang loose.

TIPS FOR PREPPING

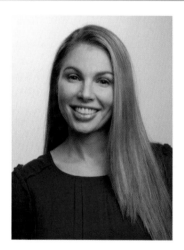 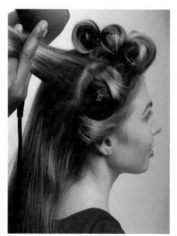 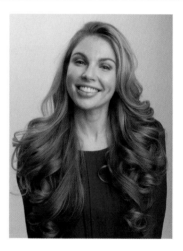

This pony looks great with straight hair or with some waves; it can even work with second-day hair. Here, hair was blow-dried with mousse and volumizing spray. Curls were added with a 1-inch curling iron and clipped in place until cool.

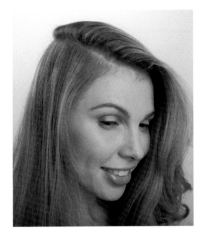

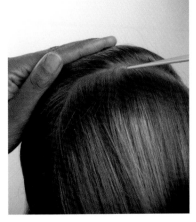

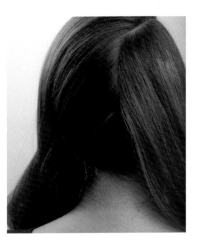

1: Brush out any curls before beginning for a more modern look. Using a rattail comb, create a deep side part. Start the part at the arch of the right eyebrow.

2: Following the shape of the head, curve the part toward the nape of the neck. Stop just behind the right ear.

3: Make a 2-inch horizontal part toward the ear to complete the section. Pin the other hair out of the way.

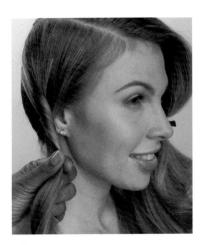

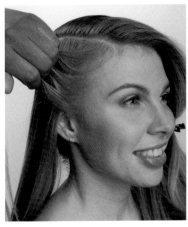

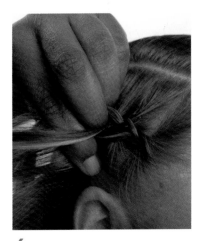

4: Sectioning should look like this. Hold the unclipped side section.

TIP: Apply holding spray after parting the hair to help keep sections separate.

5: Use a light gel to smooth the hairline. Take a small section of the right side and divide it into three strands.

6: Add anti-frizz milk to the fingertips. Begin a Dutch Braid. Cross the right strand under center, the left strand under center, and repeat. Each time hair is crossed under, pick up hair from that side.

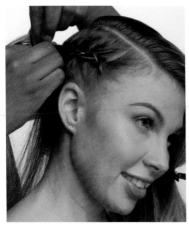

7: Continue the Dutch Braid toward the back of the head, as straight as possible. Do not follow the round shape of the scalp.

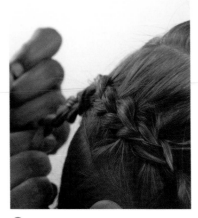

8: Once all hair has been picked up on the side, begin a Three-Strand Braid. Continue to ends.

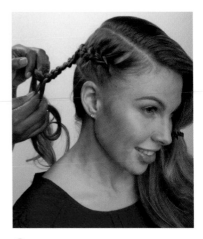

9: After completing the braid, allow it to hang free. Remove the clips holding the remaining hair.

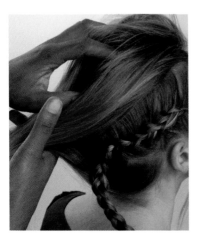

10: Sprinkle some texture powder (page 6) in the crown area. Rub the powder into the roots.

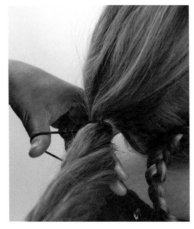

11: Gather hair into a ponytail and secure with an elastic band. Make sure to leave texture and volume in the crown.

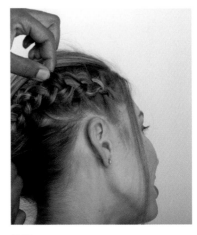

12: Use the pancaking technique to add width and texture to the braid. Gently tug the outside of each braid loop.

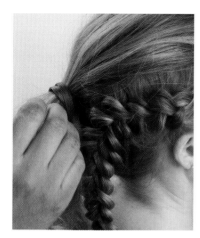 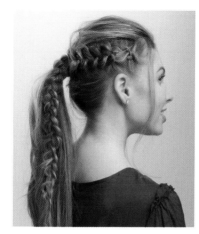

13: Take a small piece of hair from the ponytail and wrap it around the base to hide the elastic. Pin to secure.

14: Bobby pin the braid to the base of the ponytail. Finish with maximum hold hair spray.

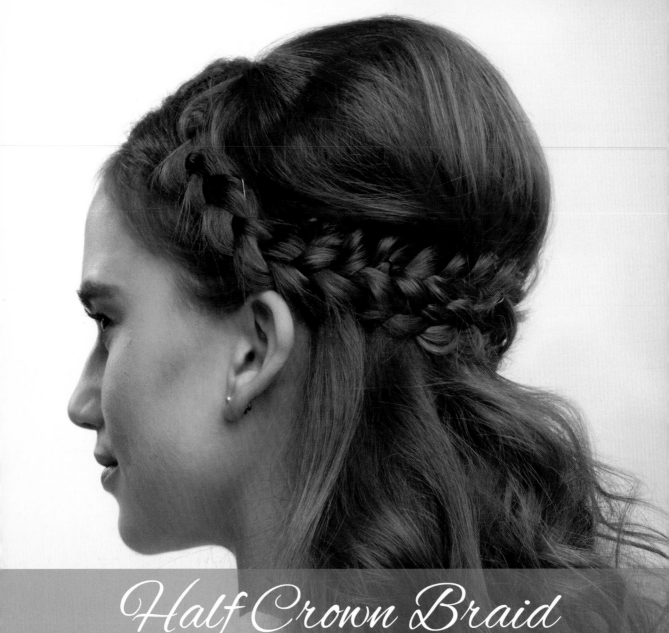

Half Crown Braid

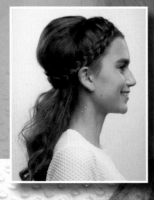

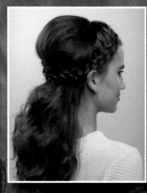

No fancy updos here—you're the type of princess who spends her days singing in the forest or daydreaming about life outside your lonely village or tower. The Half Crown Braid is great for the next ball, wedding, and formal event, but still adds some personality paired with loose, flowing locks. Luckily, you won't need too much help to master this look. I recommend starting with wavy or textured waves as a base; that way, loose hair will have some volume and texture. The super-simple, easy Dutch Braid (page 47) is the main focus of this style. It can be replaced with other braids as well, like the Basic Fishtail (page 20) or Knot Braid (page 24). However, once you've mastered these techniques, you might want to try upgrading to a more formal updo. Check out page 108 for a variation on this look fit for a queen. While I'm no fairy godmother, I promise this look can definitely outlast the last stroke of the clock at midnight.

TIPS FOR PREPPING

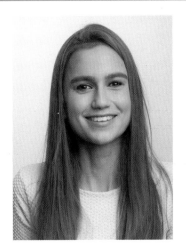 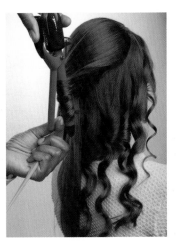 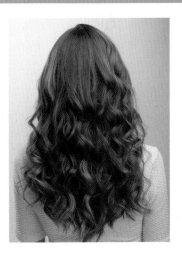

I really enjoy how waves dress up this style. To get this look, spray hair with a thermal setting spray and curl it with a ¾-inch curling iron. For a more casual look, I recommend bypassing the iron and using the hair's natural curl.

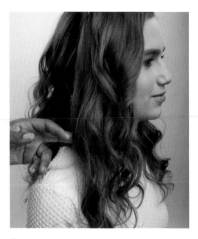 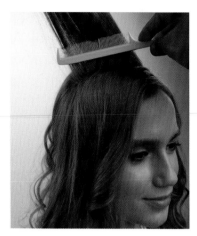 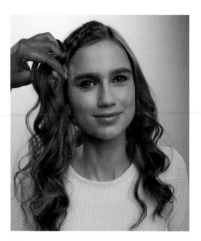

1: Create a side part starting at the arch of the left eyebrow. Create another part, horizontal, from ear to ear.

2: Backcomb the wider, right section of hair. For more manageable hair, backcomb in 1-inch-wide sections.

3: Select a small subsection from mid-crown of the right section. Divide hair into three strands. Begin a Dutch Braid. Cross the right strand under the center strand. Cross the left strand under the center strand. Pick up hair on either side each time a strand is crossed. Direct Dutch Braid toward the hairline.

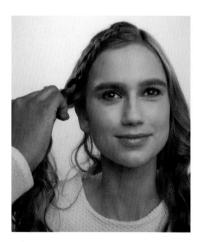 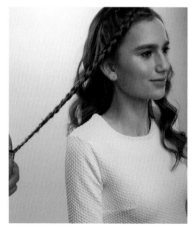 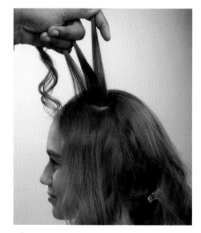

4: Once you reach the hair-line, transition to a lace braid, adding in sections only from the left side to the braid.

5: When all of the top section hair has been laced in, continue with a standard Three-Strand Braid. Secure with an elastic band.

6: On the left side, take up a small subsection of hair from mid-crown. Divide hair into three strands.

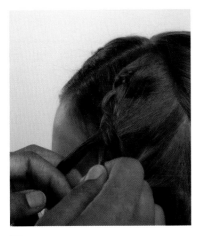

7: Begin a Dutch Braid, working toward the hairline.

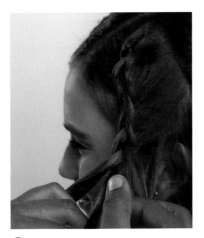

8: After reaching the hairline, transition to a lace braid. Pick up sections only from the right side of the braid.

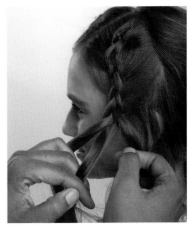

9: Once all hair has been laced in, transition to a standard Three-Strand Braid. Direct braid toward the back of the head.

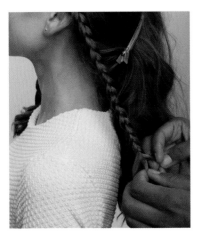

10: Continue the standard Three-Strand Braid to ends. Secure braid with an elastic braid.

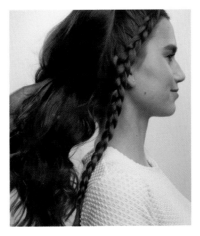

11: Sprinkle texture powder throughout the hair and on the two braids for added body.

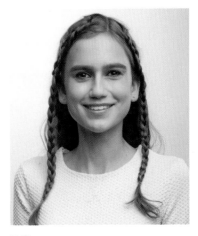

12: Let the braids hang free. The next steps will concentrate on the wavy hair in the back.

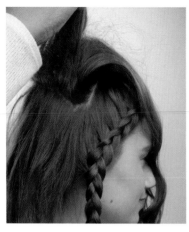

13: In 1-inch sections at the crown, hold up and back brush toward the scalp for added volume. Use a grooming brush (page 3).

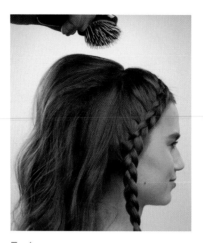

14: With the same grooming brush, smooth the top of the hair to create a natural bump, or smooth volume.

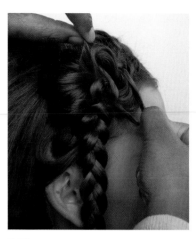

15: Gently pull on the outside loops of the Dutch Braid using the pancaking method. This creates more volume and texture. Add texture powder to the braid if needed.

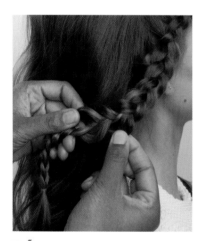

16: Continue pancaking the braid throughout its entire length. Make the braid as wide as possible.

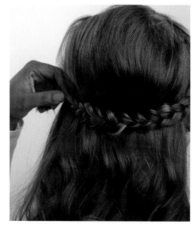

17: Take the braid from the right side and cross it over the back of the head to the left side.

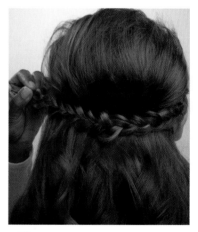

18: The braid should sit just under the bump of volume created by the back brushing. Use bobby pins to pin the braid in place. Cross the bobby pins for added security.

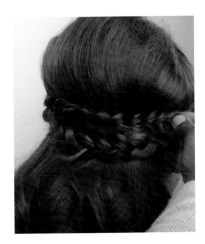

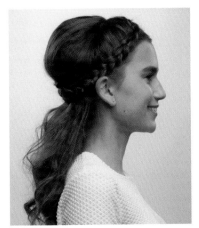

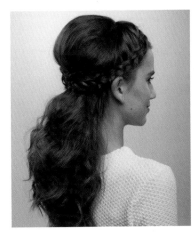

19: Cross the left braid across the back of the head. Place it above the right braid. If it's too long, tuck it underneath the right braid and flat against the head. Secure with bobby pins.

20: Fluff curls to create desired volume. If volume is uneven, simply use the tail of a comb to lift it into place.

21: Finish the look with a spray serum and holding spray.

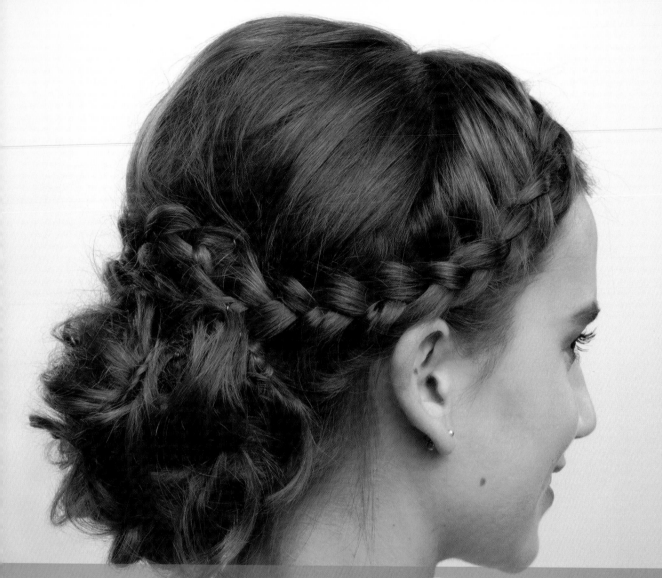

An Elegant Twist

(Variation)

For those who love the look of the Half Crown Braid (page 90), this adds a more formal touch. With this elegant variation, we'll be adding a few extra braids and twists to make the bottom of this updo just as impressive as the crown.

This style takes a little bit of work, but it's well worth the effort when it comes to formal events. This would be an amazing style for a wedding or prom.

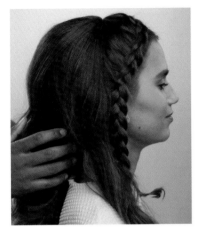

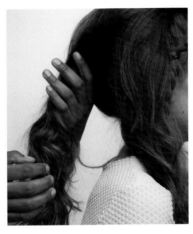

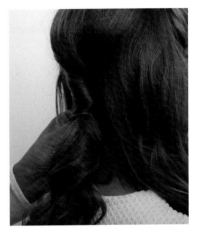

1: Follow steps 1 to 19 of the Half Crown Braid. Remove the bobby pins and release the braids. Don't unbraid the braided hair or remove volume created with the back brushing.

2: Divide the curled hair into three equal sections. Focus on the middle section.

3: Hold the middle section of hair loosely in the left hand. Twist the section to the right by turning the wrist to the left. Be careful to avoid flattening the voluminous base while twisting.

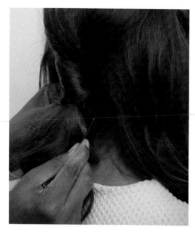

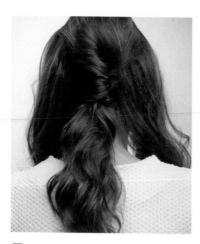

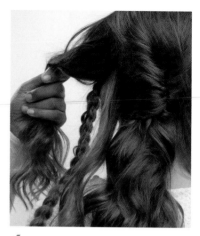

4: Slide in a long bobby pin upward from the bottom of the twist. Cross a second bobby pin to secure.

5: Allow the curly ends to hang free. This will come into play in later steps.

6: Select a 2-inch section from the bottom left section of the hair.

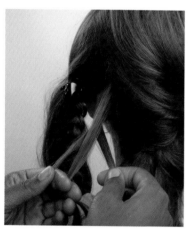

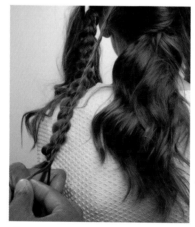

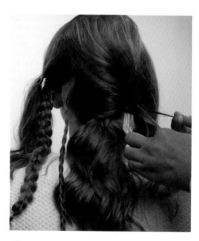

7: Clip the remaining hair on the left side out of the way. Add a little anti-frizz milk to fingertips to prep for braiding. Divide the 2-inch section into three strands. Begin a standard Three-Strand Braid, crossing the right strand over the center strand.

8: Continue the braid by crossing the left strand over the center strand. Repeat to the ends. Secure the braid with a hair-colored elastic band.

9: Repeat steps 6 to 8 on the right side.

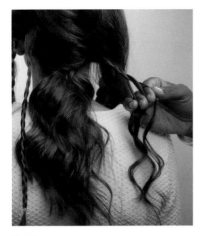

10: Secure the second three-strand brand with a hair-colored elastic band.

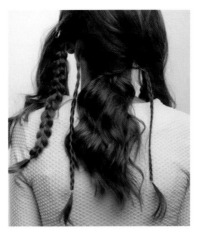

11: Let the braids hang freely. They'll be used later to style and accessorize the updo.

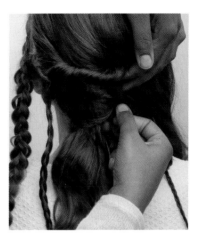

12: Twist hair from the left section toward the right side of the head. Lay the left twist over the wider center twist.

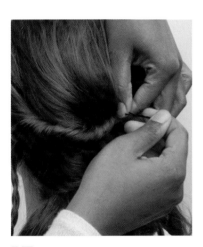

13: Pin the twist by directing the pin up into the twist, then downward into the crease of the wider twist.

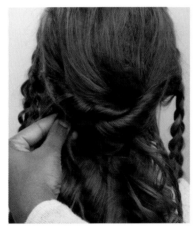

14: Repeat steps 12 and 13 with the right section of hair. Cross this second twist over the first twist.

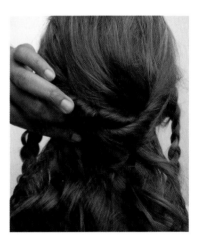

15: Cross two bobby pins to secure the twist in place. Merge the twist by directing pins upward into one twist, then downward into the other twist.

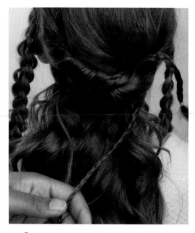

16: Move the smaller side braids out of the way for this next step.

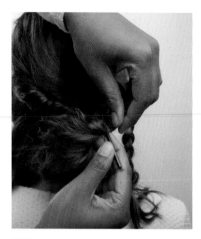

17: Hold the ends of the center section. Loosely twist clockwise, keeping curls visible. Spiral hair down toward scalp and bobby pin at the base.

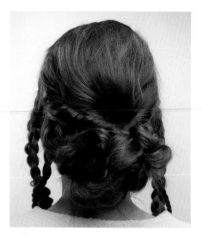

18: Repeat step 17 on the left and right sections of curls. The spiraled down sections should resemble cinnamon rolls.

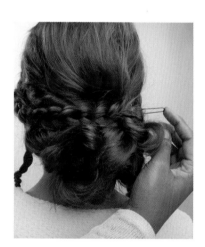

19: Use long hair pins to weave and merge the sections into a large bun. This creates a uniform look.

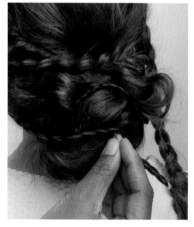

20: Cross the front left braid over the top of the twisted hair. Bobby pin braid to the right side.

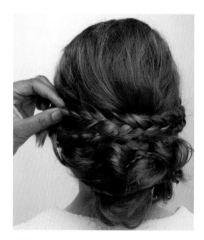

21: Weave the small braids throughout the twisted faux bun. This adds an extra bit of detail to the style.

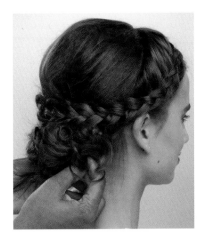

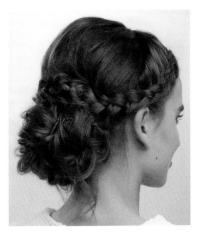

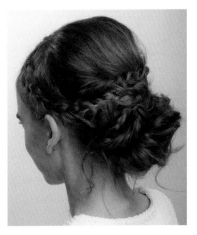

22: Cross the front right braid over, just above the left braid. If the braid is too long, tuck ends under before pinning.

23: Use hair pins to widen and shape the bun to personal preference.

24: Allow small tendrils of hair to fall loosely from the faux bun. This adds some playfulness and fun!

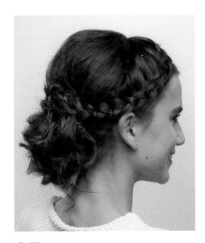

25: Use a long bobby pin to secure the faux bun close to the nape. A closer bun offers a more complete look. Finish with a spray serum and firm holding spray.

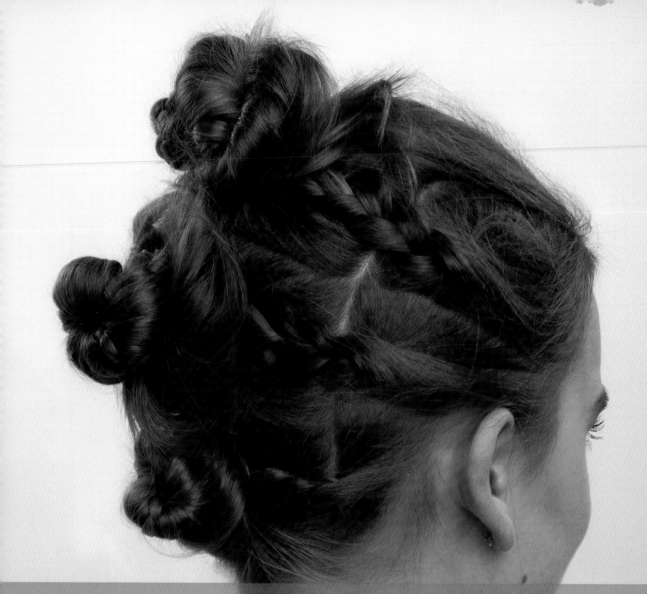

Rock-Out Style

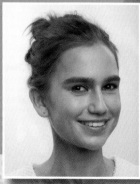
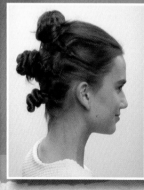
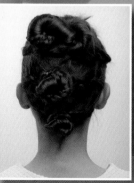

Hey there, wild child. It's time to channel that inner guitar-wielding goddess with this super-simple Rock-Out Style. A mixture of Three-Strand Braids and twisted buns create this rad, punk, chic updo that works for aspiring superstars with any hair texture. With so many cool details, this style looks complex but is actually very easy once you've mastered the art of sectioning. Sectioning is all about using your handy rattail comb to section off areas for the base of these braids. Turn it up to 11 by changing the basic braids to fishtail braids for a more detailed look. Or leave the bottom sections down and let your hair loose for a fun partial updo.

Whether you're shredding a guitar solo, crowd surfing at an outdoor festival, or hanging out backstage at the after-party, this is the ultimate rockstar look. Headbang all night—this style will outlast your most extreme thrash—but after the last encore, you'll have to take this one down before going to bed.

TIPS FOR PREPPING

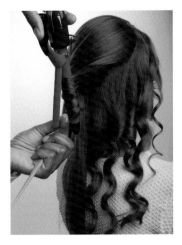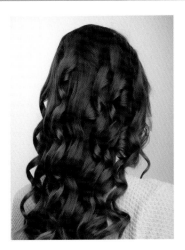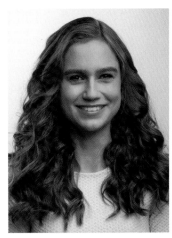

This style can be created with wet, textured, or any iron-set hair. Here, hair was blow-dried with a volumizing mousse and gel, which helps the style stay in place. Hair was then curled with a ¾-inch curling iron.

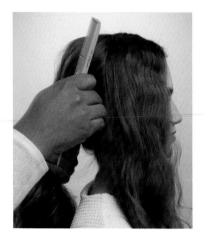

1: A rattail comb is your go-to tool in creating the most important part of this style: the sections.

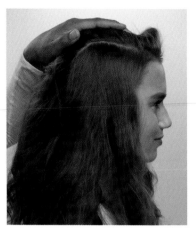

2: Begin sectioning by parting from the inside corner of the right eyebrow straight back to the nape of the neck.

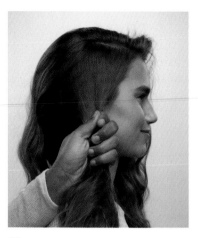

3: Clip bottom section of hair out of way. Repeat sectioning from step 2 on the left side of the head.

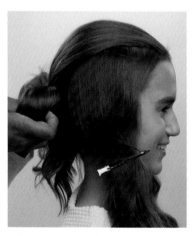

4: This creates a "Mohawk" section on the top of the head. Gather the center Mohawk into a ponytail.

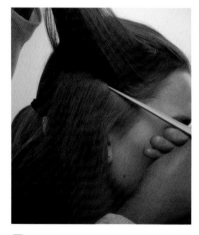

5: Using the rattail comb, add two horizontal partings on the right side. This will divide the hair into 3 sections.

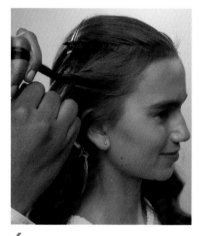

6: Begin a Three-Strand Braid with the top section. Start the braid midway back, closer to the center of the head.

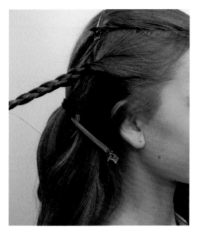

7: Continue the Three-Strand Braid to the ends of the hair. Secure with an elastic band and pin out of the way.

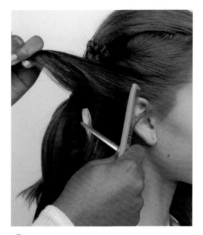

8: Comb through the second section, which should be just behind the ear, to prep. Begin a Three-Strand Braid with this section.

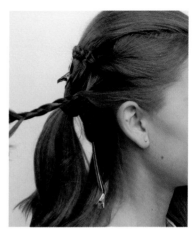

9: Continue braiding to ends and secure with an elastic band.

TIP: Use a serum or anti-frizz milk to avoid frizz while braiding.

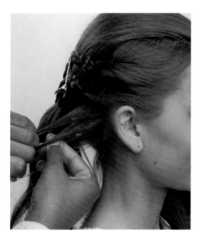

10: Smooth the third section at the nape of the neck to keep it neat and prep for braiding.

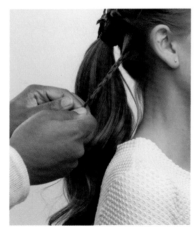

11: Create a Three-Strand Braid in this third section. Continue to ends and secure with an elastic braid.

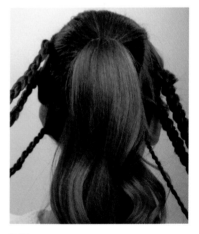

12: Repeat steps 5 through 11 on the right side of the head. When you are done, there should be 6 braids.

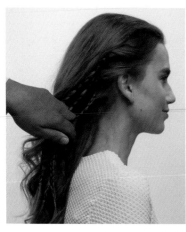 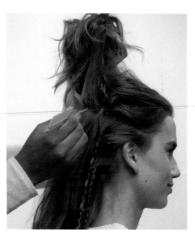 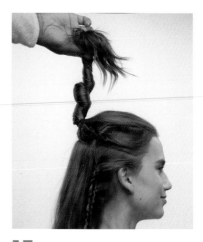

13: Release the center Mohawk section. It's time to create some magic!

14: Section an area at the top of the head. Follow the horizontal partings from the upper side sections to create a part, connecting the right side to the left.

15: Gather the top section and top braids from both sides into a ponytail. Secure with an elastic band. Twist the ponytail repeatedly.

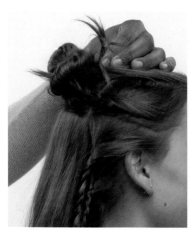 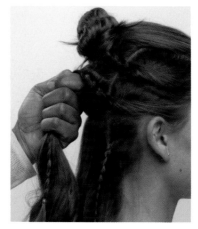 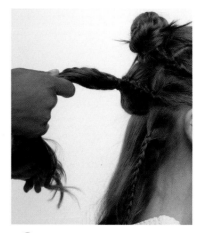

16: Twist hair down into a figure 8. Pin in place with long bobby pins or hair pins. Leave the ends free.

17: Create a second section by following and connecting the horizontal side parts from left to right.

18: Gather this second section and two outside center braids into a ponytail. Secure with an elastic band.

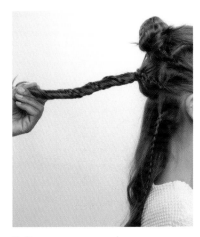

19: Twist the ponytail down into the shape of a cinnamon roll. Secure with bobby pins.

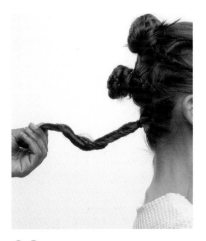

20: Gather bottom section and outside braids into a ponytail. Secure with an elastic band.

TIP: Smooth bottom hairline toward ponytail for a finished look.

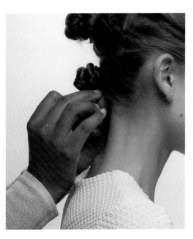

21: Twist the final section into a bun and secure with bobby pins.

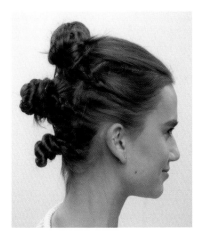

22: Time to rock 'n' roll! Finish the style with maximum hold hair spray.

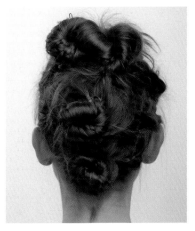

23: To add more texture and that runway-chic look, sprinkle texture powder into hands and rub palm of hands over the braids.

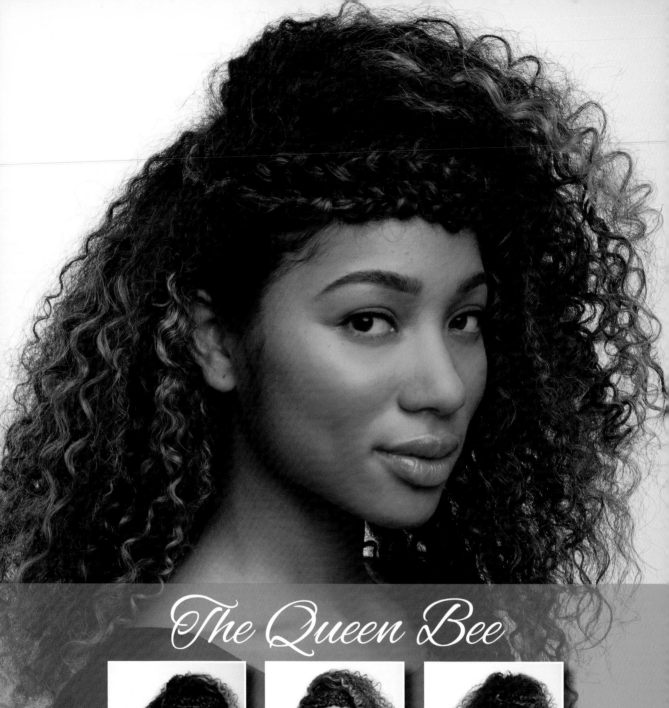

The Queen Bee

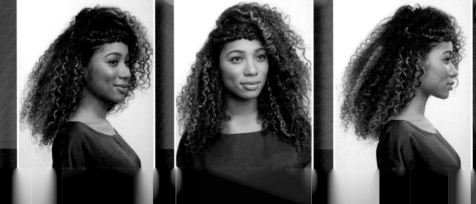

Who runs the world? You do. Especially with this everyday look that blends edgy and regal. Two simple Three-Strand Braids act as this style's base and create a crown-like headband that frames the face while allowing the rest of your locks to flow free. This funky style is a great way to spice up typically loose hair, perfect when you're on the go but still want to impress your subjects. The Three-Strand Braids make this an easy style for beginners.

The Queen Bee works for any hair texture, although I love the way more textured hair gives this look a more dramatic flair. For variations on this style, try mixing it up by crossing braids in the back of the head or even on one side instead of in the front. Never fear, your crown won't fall apart until you're ready to loosen this braid. Wherever you go, you'll be sure to make a royal entrance with this simple style.

TIPS FOR PREPPING

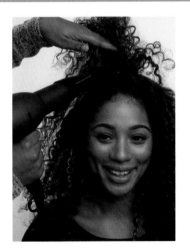 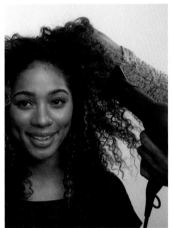 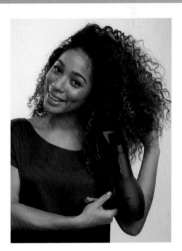

Prep damp, freshly shampooed hair with a leave-in conditioner and gel or mousse. This model used a leave-in conditioner, light styling moisturizer, and light gel recommended for curly hair. Let hair air dry, or blow-dry to speed up the drying process. To blow-dry, use hair dryer at medium heat with a diffuser attachment to direct heat. Tilt head to the side and hold the dryer at least 8 inches away while drying. Don't touch hair until dry to avoid frizz.

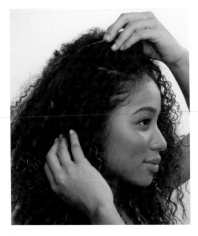

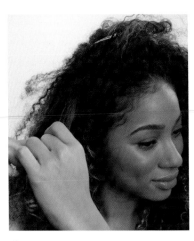

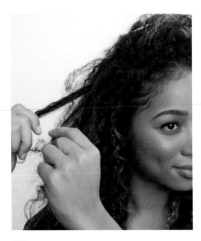

1: Create a deep side part on one side of the head. The part should be at least 3 inches wide.

2: Clip hair section on top. Pick up a 1-inch-wide section of hair at the back of the side parting.

3: Clip hair remaining hair below part out of way. In section 2 begin a Dutch braid to help braid lay flat.

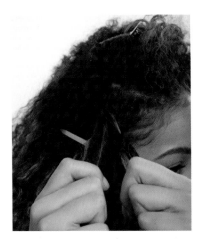

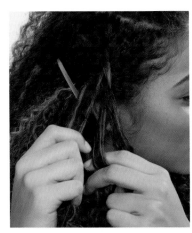

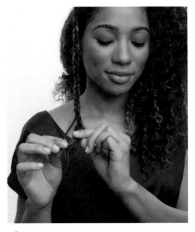

4: Instead of braiding straight down the hair shaft, direct the braid toward the opposite side of head.

5: Continue to create a Three-Strand Braid down the entire length of the hair.

6: Secure the end of hair with a rubber band or an elastic band.

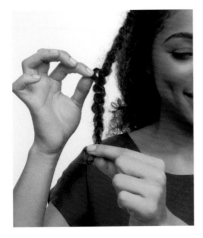

7: Pancake the braid by pulling gently on the outside edges of the braid to widen it.

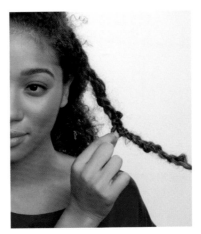

8: Complete steps 1 to 6 on the opposite side of the head. This will result in a mirror Three-Strand Braid. Be sure to pancake the braid for fullness and texture.

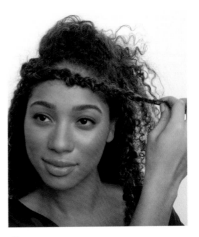

9: Take the end of the first braid across the forehead and pin to the opposite side of the head.

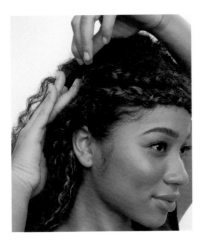

10: Repeat step 9 with the second braid, placing the opposite braid above the first braid.

TIP: Place a bobby pin into the elastic band for securing the first braid into the base of the second braid.

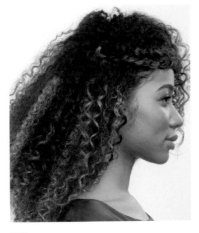

11: Pin the braids together to avoid a gap between braids. This makes the braids appear very full.

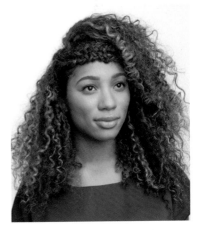

12: Fluff up textured hair on top and direct most to one side. This shows off the cute braided crown.

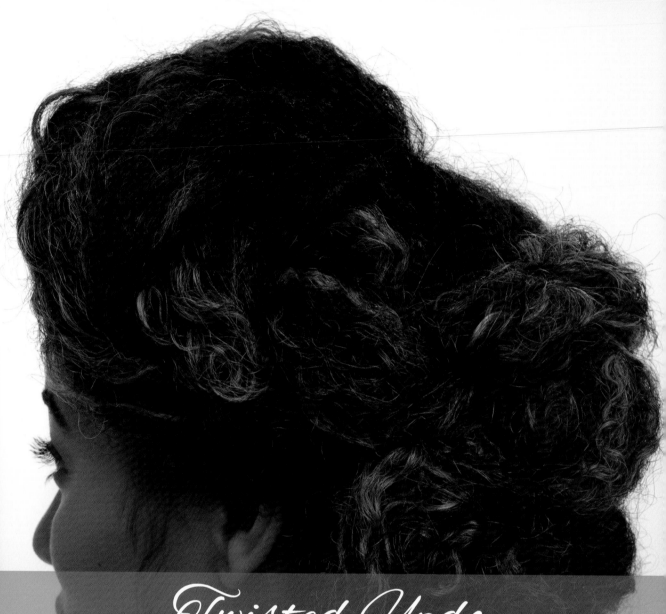

Twisted Updo

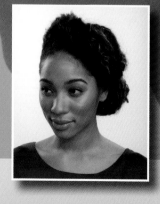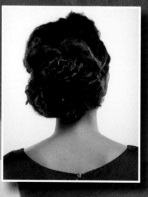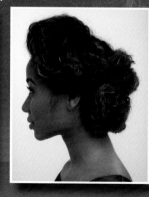

Calling all my curly haired lovelies—the Twisted Updo was designed with you in mind. This is great for anyone with thick and textured hair. All that extra volume and structure is absolutely crucial for adding an intricate and elegant look. And did I mention that this style is amazingly easy?! Easy from start to finish, this look only uses two different sections and a variation of twists.

The twist (and its variations) is the style sister of the braid and perfect for beginners. We'll introduce the flat twist, Two-Strand Twist, and Three-Strand Twist. If you want to keep it even simpler, I would totally recommend trying this look with just one type of twist as well. If you want to level up, try out a Dutch Braid (page 47) or Basic Fishtail (page 20) in the place of any of the twists.

Simple and stylish, this style is the perfect way to tame that mane while making a splash at formal events, like weddings or the prom. This updo is completely secure; you'll be set to dance all night, curly girl.

TIPS FOR PREPPING

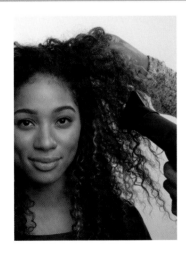 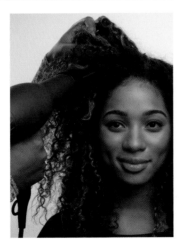 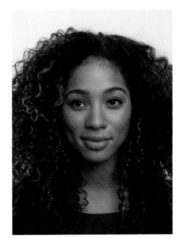

For this style, gel for curly hair was applied to wet, natural curls. Curls were defused as they dried. Defined curls help the entire look come together at the end. Generally, it's important that curls are well-defined for any curly hairstyle.

If hair isn't naturally curly, consider applying tight Dutch Braids or three-strand twists to wet hair. Allow strands to dry overnight and then remove braids, resulting in a similar curl set.

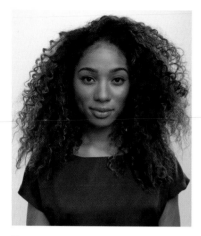

1: Begin with moisturized and well-defined curls.

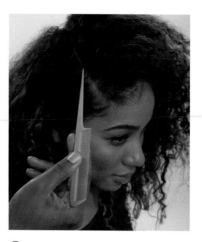

2: Create an L-shaped section, parting from the arch of the right eyebrow and pushing hair back and across to the front of the left ear.

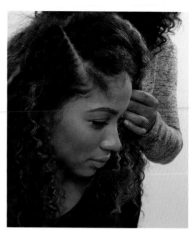

3: Clip this section of hair, including fringe or bangs, out of the way.

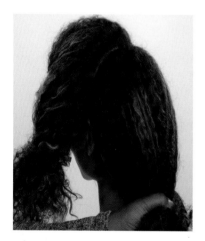

4: This style is very easy to achieve because it only involves two sections. Add anti-frizz milk or serum to both sections to minimize frizz.

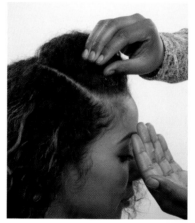

5: Apply a strong-hold gel or mousse to smooth down hair at the hairline. Make sure to smooth hair at the nape of the neck as well.

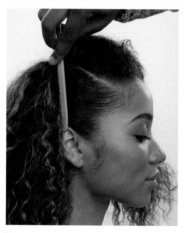

6: Using a rattail comb or a brush, smooth down the hairline. Direct the right section away from the face.

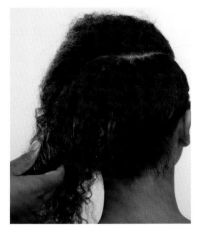

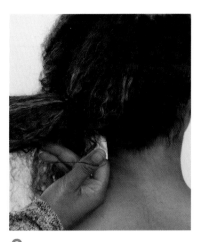

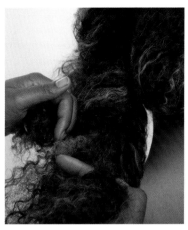

7: Beginning behind the right ear, take the bottom section, roll it, and tuck it downward toward the nape of the neck, directing it toward the left ear. This creates a flat twist that will become the base of this style.

8: Once hair reaches the left side, hold it tightly and secure with an elastic band to create a ponytail.

9: Divide the ponytail into 3 sections. Begin a Three-Strand Twist (page 38).

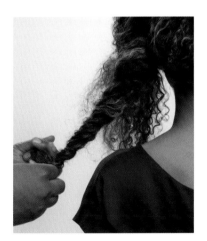

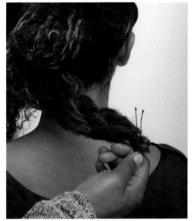

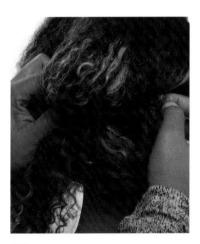

10: Continue until you reach the ends of the hair and the Three-Strand Twist is complete.

11: Flip the ends over to make a loop. Secure with an elastic band. Place a bobby pin in the loop.

12: Cross the Three-Strand Twist to from the left to the right side and secure with the bobby pin at the base of the flat twist, behind the right ear.

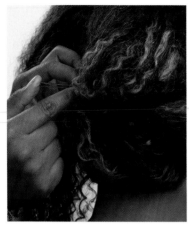

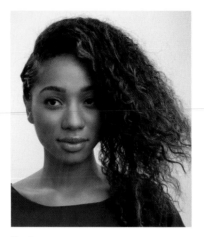

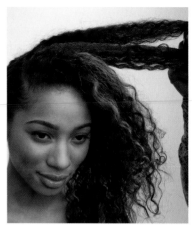

13: With a simple twist, we've created what looks to be a complex style! Use hair pins to merge the Three-Strand Twist with the flat twist. Gently tug on any loop to add width and texture.

14: Smooth the hairline of the top section with gel. Brush hair way from the face.

15: Take two sections from the back of the top section. Start a laced Two-Strand Twist by placing the right strand over the left.

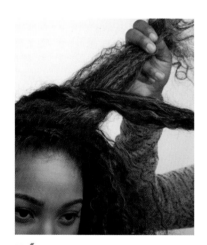

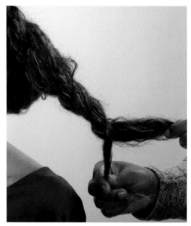

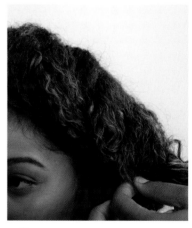

16: Continue right over left. Pick up hair each time the left strand crosses under the right strand.

17: Continue twisting right, only picking up hair from the left side. Continue this laced Two-Strand Twist to ends.

18: Gently tug on each section of the twist to add fullness and show off those beautiful defined curls.

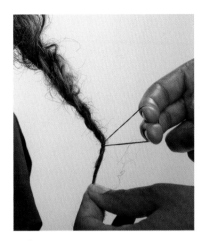

19: Secure ends with an elastic band.

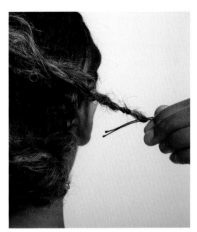

20: Fold the ends of the twist over to create a loop. Place a bobby pin into the loop and pin the hair to the right side of the twists in the back.

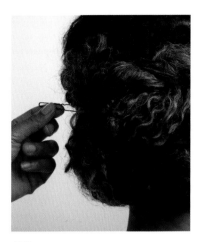

21: Using hair pins, merge loops of the twist together and merge any gaps in the hair. This makes the style appear more polished.

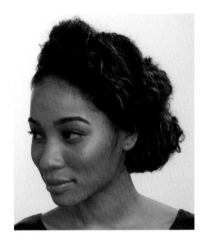

22: Gently tug any sections of the hair to widen and create balance within the style. Finish this look with a spray serum.

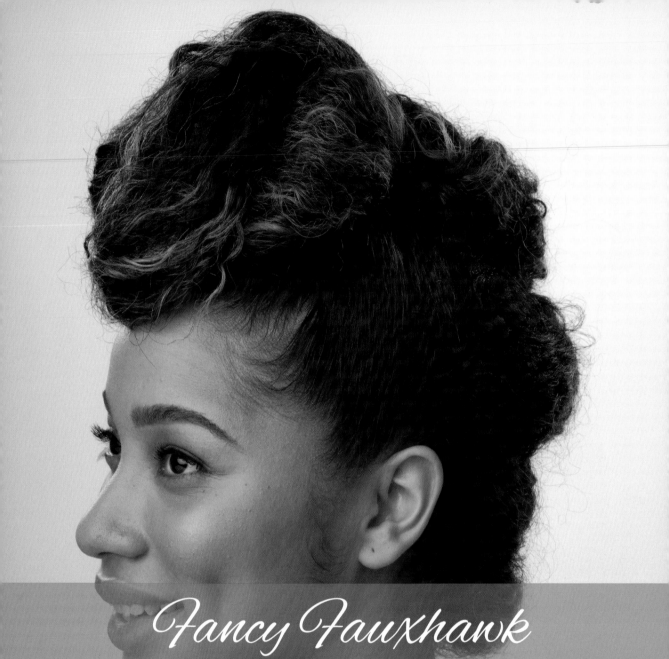

Fancy Fauxhawk

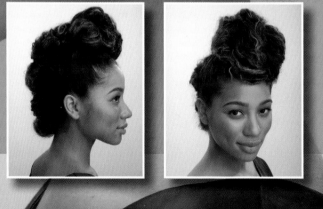

Always wanted a Mohawk, but could never commit? Today's your lucky day. You can finally get that edgy look, but with an extremely modern and elegant twist. Appropriate for any event where you want to be the center of attention, whether it's a rock concert or a night at the symphony, the Fancy Fauxhawk is all about attitude.

You can get this big-hair look easily. With some easy sectioning, two simple Three-Strand Twists, and a few carefully placed hair pins, this look can be done in a few minutes by even the most beginner-level braiders. Plus, the hair pins will really secure the style throughout the night. Try this style on curly or frizzy hair textures, as they will have the volume and texture that really makes this style stunning. If an updo isn't fitting your mood for the night, try leaving the bottom two sections down for a cool and casual partial updo.

TIPS FOR PREPPING

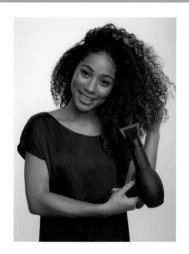 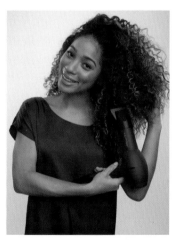 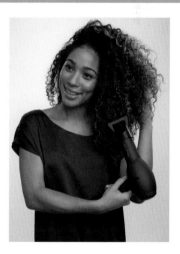

Use natural curls with this look. Defuse them with a light gel specifically geared toward defining ringlets. To create your own ringlets and curls, set wet hair with Three-Strand Braids, twists, or braids. Once they're dry, release the braids with serum on the fingertips.

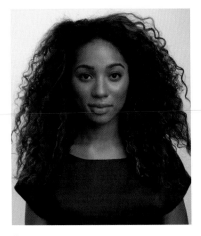

1: Start this style with freshly defined curls and ringlets, or second-day curls.

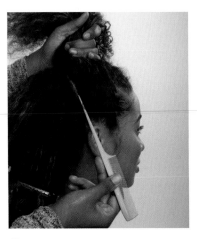

2: With a rattail comb, create a horizontal part from ear to ear, separating the front and back portion of hair.

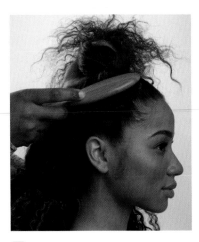

3: Add gel to the hairline. With a soft bristle brush, smooth the hairline. Gather a ponytail with the top section.

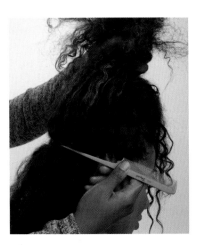

4: Divide the remaining hair in half by creating a horizontal part from the top of one ear to the other.

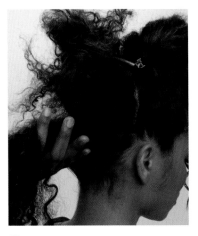

5: Use a duckbill clip to secure the midsection out of way. The next steps will work with the bottom section.

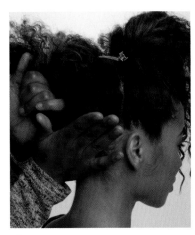

6: Add gel to the hairline.

TIP: Use the palm of your hand to smooth the hairline before brushing it smooth.

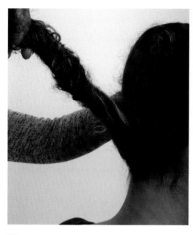

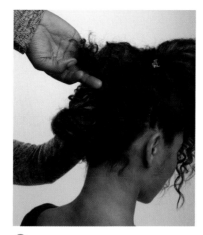

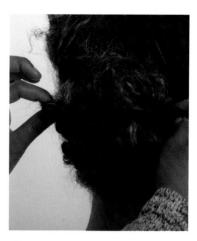

7: Gather the bottom section of hair into one hand. Twist to the left from root to tip.

8: Twist the hair down on itself, into a bun, toward the scalp.

9: After twisting hair down into a bun, use long bobby pins to hold the section down. Once pinned, gently tug on the outside of the twist to widen the bun.

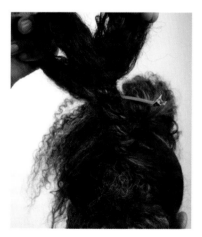

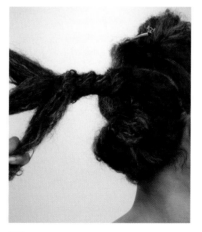

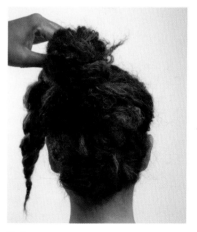

10: Release the midsection from the clip. Add gel to the hairline and brush smooth. It's important to keep the edges neat for this style. Divide this section into three strands.

11: Create a Three-Strand Twist (page 38). Cross the center strand over the right strand, cross the left strand all the way over the right strand. Repeat. Finish at ends with a few stitches of a Three-Strand Braid.

12: Repeat steps 10 and 11 with the top section of hair.

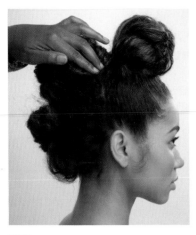

13: Roll the center section up and down to the scalp. Mirror the height of the bottom twist and secure with bobby pins.

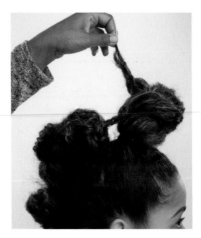

14: Repeat with the top section, rolling up and pinning. Pin the end of the top twist into the middle twist.

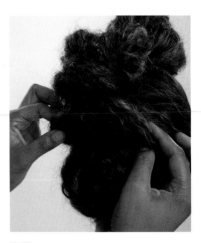

15: Gently tug on the center section to widen the twist. This offers a more wearable style.

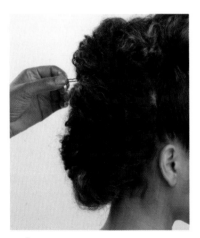

16: Use hair pins to merge the three twists together.

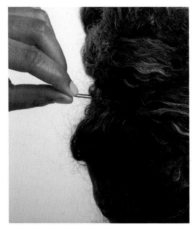

17: Cover any gaps between the twists. Concentrate on covering the parts that separate the sections.

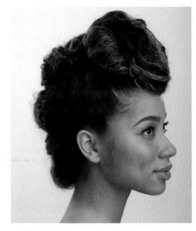

18: Check the balance of the style, making sure that the height of all the twists are consistent. Finish the look with a spray serum and holding spray.

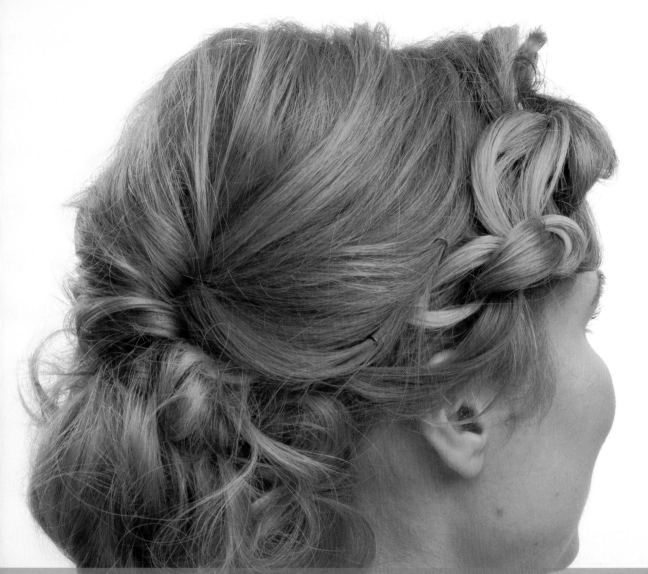

The Knotted Updo

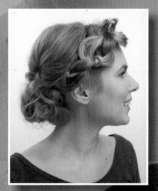

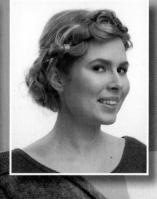

Looking for an all-night updo that won't take all day to put together? The Knotted Updo is your solution. This very simple style takes one of the easiest braid techniques, the Knot Braid (page 24), and adds a few twists to make a really elegant updo in a matter of minutes. You can be an absolute beginner, yet completely handle doing hair for prom or fancy dinners. All you need is a few elastic bands and a handful of pins.

For this style, channel some of that creativity! I recommend using smooth, straight, or slightly wavy hair for this style. The knots that frame the face will have the most detail with polished and silky hair. If you do have waves (either from a curling iron or your natural wave), you can try leaving the back of the hair down as a partial updo. Even though it is a simple braid, it is pretty sturdy and will last throughout a fun night of dancing.

TIPS FOR PREPPING

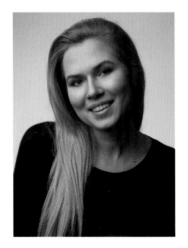 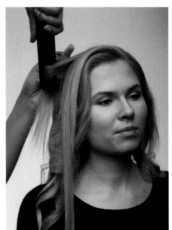 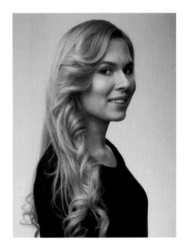

For this updo, create curls to smooth the hair and add texture. Both will help to work with the hair. To start, blow-dry hair with a round brush with mousse and a thermal setting spray. Use a 1-inch flat iron to create loose curls.

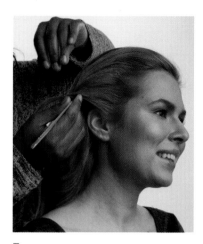

1: Brush all hair to the back.

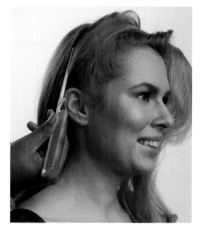

2: Use a rattail comb to create a section, starting from behind the right ear and ending behind the left ear.

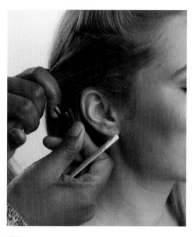

3: Make a horizontal section 2 inches above the ear. Clip hair out of the way with a duckbill clip.

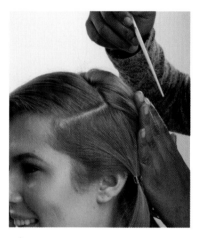

4: Repeat step 3 on the other side of the head.

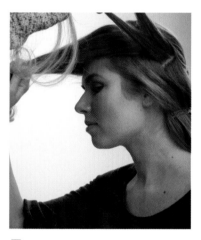

5: Take a 1-inch section from the back left area of the crown section. Divide hair from this section into two strands.

TIP: Apply anti-frizz milk to fingertips to reduce flyaways.

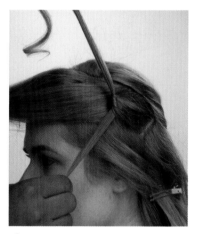

6: Cross the left strand over, then under the right strand and through the hole. Pull to tighten down to the scalp. This is just like tying a shoe! If needed, adjust the knot and smooth strands with serum.

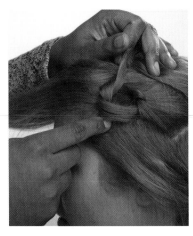

7: While holding the two strands, pick up another 1-inch-wide section of hair from the top section. Divide the 1-inch section into two and add to the current strands. Repeat knot braid from 6.

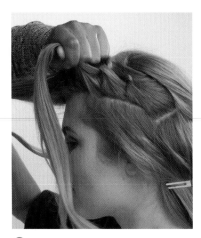

8: Repeat 7 with another 1-inch section.

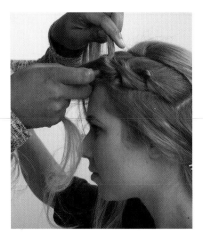

9: At this point, the knot pattern is developing. Make sure that each knot is in the same direction (left over and under right) to avoid tangling.

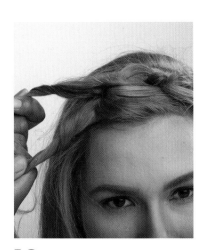

10: Continue the knot braid, picking up 1-inch sections and crossing left strand over, then under the right strand.

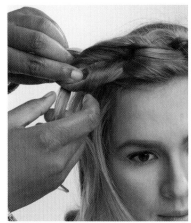

11: For extra detail and texture, twist the two strands in opposite directions. Twisting the hair will also offer extra volume at the hairline.

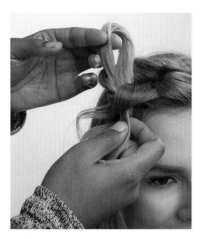

12: Continue the knot braid with another 1-inch section of hair.

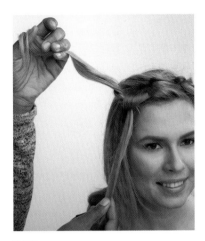

13: Gently pull on the two strands to tighten the knots to the scalp.

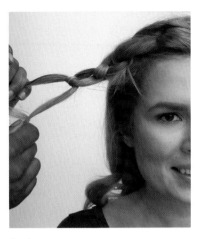

14: Once all hair from the top section is picked up, continue creating knots to ends. Secure with an elastic band.

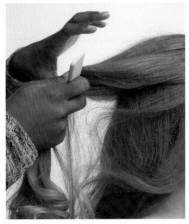

15: Release side sections. Create a horizontal part from the left ear to the right ear, allowing it to join the horizontal part created earlier.

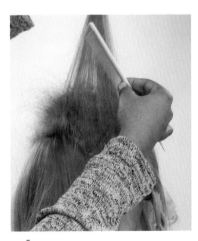

16: Hold the top section of hair straight up. Using a rattail comb, push hair toward the scalp to create volume.

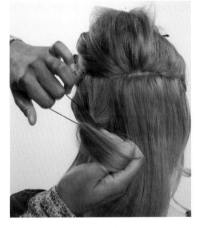

17: Pin the top section out of the way. Create two even ponytails from the bottom section of hair.

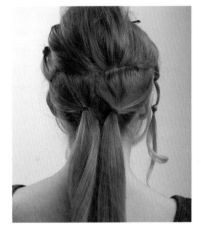

18: Make the base of the ponytails as close as possible. This technique creates more texture in the ponytail.

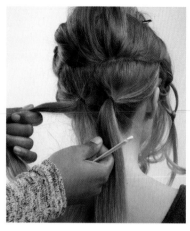

19: Divide the left ponytail into two even strands.

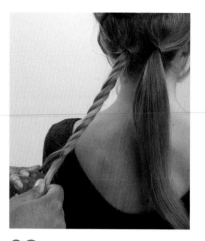

20: Create a Two-Strand Twist. Twist the left strand over the right. Then, the right strand under the left. Repeat to ends.

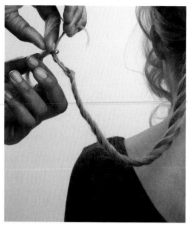

21: Secure the twist with an elastic band.

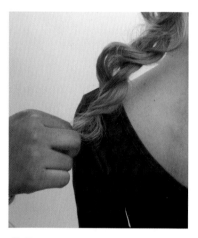

22: Starting at the bottom of the twist, while holding on to one of the strands, push the other strand up toward the scalp to create volume and texture. Repeat steps 19 to 22 with the right twist.

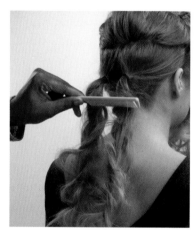

23: Place the rattail comb within the twist and push the hair toward the scalp. Do this multiple times throughout the length of the twists.

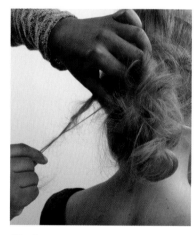

24: Gather both twists in one hand and twist counter clockwise to create a messy bun. Hold the hair in place and secure to the head with long bobby pins and hair pins.

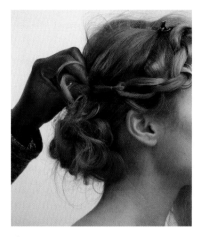

25: Bring the knotted section of hair around the right side and bobby pin it to the top of the messy bun.

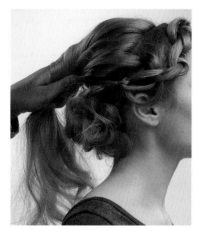

26: Unpin the top, back-combed section of the hair. Make sure not to disturb the backcombing.

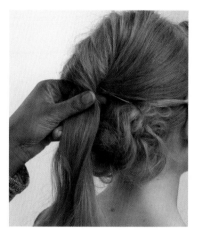

27: Gather into a ponytail above the bun and twist to the right. Bobby pin to the top of the messy bun.

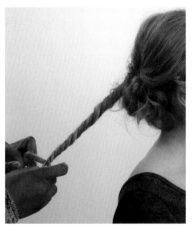

28: Once the hair is bobby pinned, pinch out some of the hair to create width. With the length of the hair, create a Two-Strand Twist.

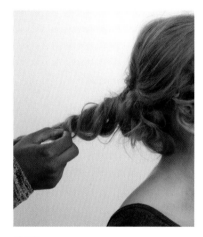

29: Hold on to one of the strands of the newly created twist. Gently push the other strand up toward the scalp to create volume and texture.

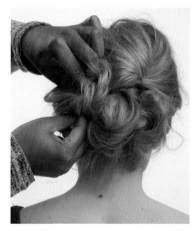

30: Roll the twist down toward the scalp into a circle shape. Pin hair toward the left of the head.

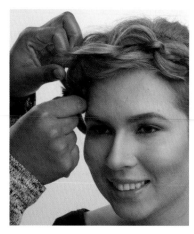 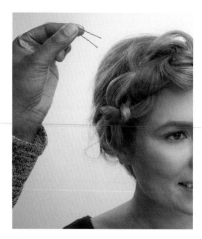 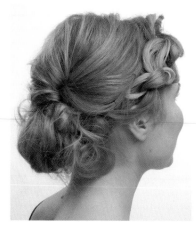

31: Go through the style and gently tug on each loop for even more volume and width. This is especially important for the hair within the knots.

32: Once sections are expanded, use small hair pins to cover any holes and gaps in the style. Finish with a light holding spray.

33: Thanks to its messy, bohemian style, this crown is a ton of fun and can last you all day.

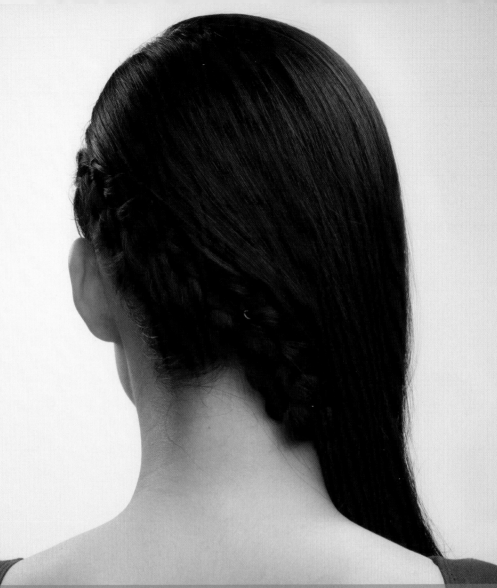

Vintage Wave Cheat

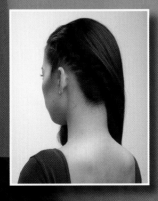
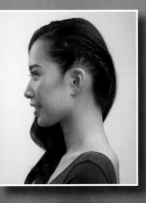
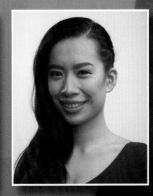

Watch out for the paparazzi, with this style you'll be channeling classic Hollywood with a modern twist. The beauty of the Vintage Wave Cheat is that it's not only glamorous, but also outrageously easy. A simple Dutch Braid behind the left ear adds a trendy detail to these yesteryear-inspired waves, creating a captivating look from any angle. For different variations on this style, try your hand at replacing the braid with a French or fishtail braid. Straight and wavy hair work best with this technique.

You'll have that red carpet appeal wherever you go with the Vintage Wave Cheat, making it ideal for formal events, dances, or a night out on the town. Don't worry about your close-up—you can expect this braid to look great and hold tight all night.

TIPS FOR PREPPING

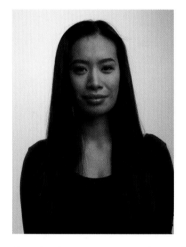 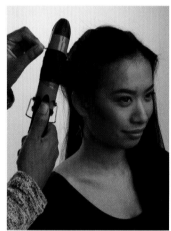 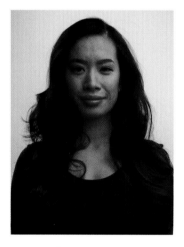

For the loose waves in this style, curl hair with a 1¼-inch curling iron. Before curling, blow-dry hair with a leave-in conditioner, mousse, and thermal setting spray. Clip curls in place to cool. This prep can be skipped if waves aren't desired.

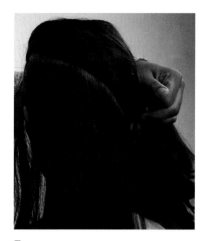

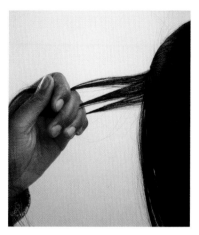

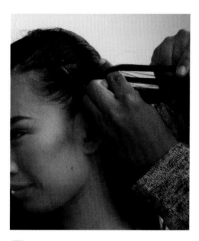

1: Part from the left temple to the back of the right ear. Secure section with a duckbill clip.

2: Apply anti-frizz milk to bottom section of hair to smooth flyaways. Take a small section near the temple, separate it into three strands, and begin a Dutch Braid (page 47).

3: While braiding, add hair from the left side of the head to the strand currently on the left side of the braid.

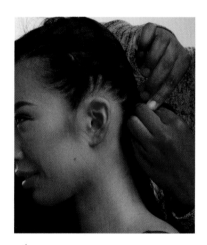

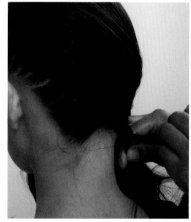

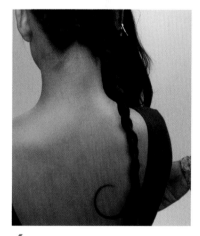

4: Continue across the back of the head, directing toward the back of the right ear.

5: Continue the Dutch Braid until you reach the right side.

TIP: Braid as close to the part as possible to help braid flow with the waves.

6: Finish with a Three-Strand Braid down the shaft of the hair. Secure with an elastic band, leaving the ends free.

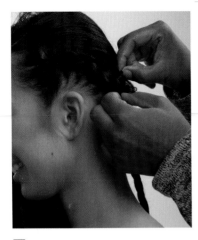

7: Widen or pancake the braid by gently pulling on the outside of each braided loop.

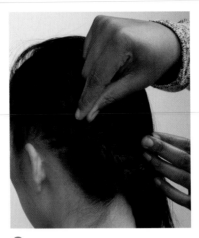

8: Bobby pin top section of hair into the braid. This makes the braid more visible and the style flow together.

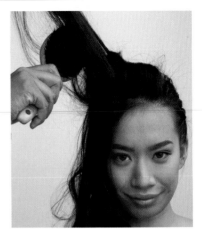

9: Back brush curls at the root to create a base. Place brush slightly above the root and push downward.

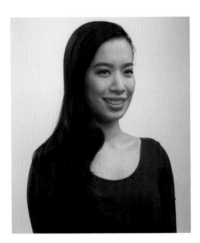

10: Once base is complete, spray hair with holding spray. Smooth hair into vintage waves.

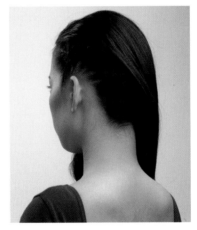

11: Make sure that hair is pinned into the braid. Lay all hair over right shoulder to complete the style.

Index

Acknowledgments

I'd like to thank my mother, Trina, for your continued love and support. Next up, my siblings Takahya, Ronnie, Akeia, and Shadia. I appreciate you all answering those late-night calls and texts, and helping me throughout life, in general. Your support means the entire world to me. Thank you to my stepfather, Lawrence, brother-in-law, Tony, and my two nephews, Amir and James. To my father, Ronnie Everett, you are loved and missed. Thank you for the support of my extended family and friends.

Major thanks to Keith Riegert for believing in me and giving me this amazing opportunity. I won't let you down. Thank you to Casie Vogel and Kourtney Joy for helping me to find my voice. Thank you to my amazing assistants, talented photographers, makeup artist, and the lovely models. I could not have done this without you. Thank you to the sponsors for providing amazing products and tools.

About the Author

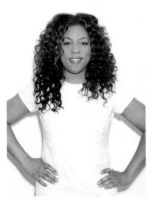

Whether sleek, sophisticated, or fashion, hairdresser **Monaé Everett** knows how to bring out the beauty in everyone. Monaé has been fortunate enough to create beautiful hairstyles for some of Hollywood's leading ladies, including Jessica Lowndes, Taraji P. Henson, Mariah Carey, and more. Her expert opinion has been featured in major publications such as *Huffington Post*, Redbook.com, and *Essence* magazine. To help make women look and feel their best, she regularly blogs at HairandMakeupBlog.com and uploads beauty tutorials to YouTube. Having had the honor of working with celebrities, styling for movies, and leading shows for New York Fashion Week, Monaé is just getting started.